Caregiving

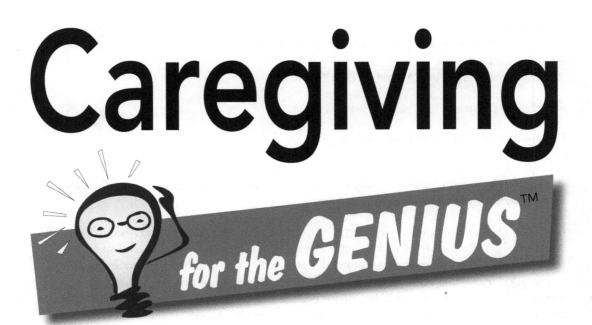

for the GENIUS™

Understand the Journey from the Inside Out

FOR THE GENIUS IN ALL OF US™

Jane W. Barton, MTS, MASM

Caregiving for the GENIUS™

One of the **For the GENIUS™** books

Published by
For the GENIUS Press, an imprint of CharityChannel LLC
30021 Tomas, Suite 300
Rancho Santa Margarita, CA 92688-2128 USA

forthegenius.com

First Edition
Library of Congress Control Number: 2013956453
ISBN Print Book: 978-1-941050-02-6 | ISBN eBook: 978-1-941050-03-3

Printed in the United States of America
10 9 8 7 6 5 4 3 2

This and most For the GENIUS Press books are available at special quantity discounts for bulk purchases for sales promotions, premiums, fundraising, or educational use. For information, contact CharityChannel, 30021 Tomas, Suite 300, Rancho Santa Margarita, CA 92688-2128 USA. +1 949-589-5938

Publisher's Acknowledgments

This book was produced by a team dedicated to excellence; please send your feedback to Editors@ForTheGENIUS.com.

Members of the team who produced this book include:

Editors

Acquisitions Editor: Linda Lysakowski

Comprehensive Editor: Linda Lysakowski

Copy Editor: Jill McLain

Production

Layout Editor: Jill McLain

Book Design: Deborah Perdue

Illustrations: Kimberly Domingo

Administrative

For the GENIUS Press: Stephen Nill, CEO, CharityChannel LLC

Marketing and Public Relations: John Millen

J ane W. Barton is a passionate speaker, writer, and listener. Jane is the founder of Cardinal, LLC, a consulting firm that provides educational programs, books, and blogs to assist people in confronting the daunting challenges posed by aging, serious illness, and end-of-life care. Jane is well versed in the areas of aging, grief and bereavement, caregiving, hospice and palliative care, change and transition, and spirituality and health. She presents innovative, transformational programs to community members, health care providers, pastoral caregivers, clergy, funeral service providers, and national audiences to improve the experience of people and families challenged by serious, advanced, or terminal illnesses.

Jane is a frequent speaker at state, regional, and national conferences pertaining to hospice and palliative care, death and dying, and aging. She serves as a national trainer for the Society of Certified Senior Advisors. Additionally, she routinely offers programs throughout her home state of Colorado for professionals and community members.

Prior to the *flight* of Cardinal, LLC, Jane served as Director of Education for a palliative care educational institute. She also served as a hospice chaplain and bereavement facilitator in hospice and palliative care. Jane is a certified Spiritual Director as well as a Certified Senior Advisor. In a former life, she worked as a financial services representative and an exploration petroleum geologist and manager.

Dedication

To Mom, the Cardinal spirit who taught me how to listen, to love, and to live.

Author's Acknowledgments

Writing is a solitary activity; however, a book is the result of creative collaboration. So I would like to express my heartfelt gratitude to my esteemed colleagues, cherished friends, and beloved family who helped in the birthing of this book. I couldn't have done this without you!

I want to thank Frank, a colleague and friend, for the gracious introduction to Linda Lysakowski, my editor. The introduction led to the realization of a lifelong dream—writing and publishing a book. Linda is an editor *extraordinaire;* she improves the final product while honoring and retaining the author's voice. Thank you, Linda.

I'm also incredibly thankful for the honest assessments, insights, and suggestions provided by those who read the manuscript prior to publication: Kay, Stacie, Cheryl, JoAnne, David, Cynthia, Morie, Richard, Jeanne, Chris, Frank, Rick, Jamie, and Susan. A special note of thanks goes to my dear friend Kay, who provided timely and specific commentary throughout the writing process. To one and all, thank you for providing the needed spit and polish.

We learn best through the lived experience, the stories. So this book is filled with stories intended to educate, inspire, and challenge. Thus, I want to thank the people who touched my life in memorable ways and contributed to the composite stories. I learned at the feet of some incredible spirits. Their stories will benefit you as well.

To my family, my eternal love and gratitude. Writing is an all-consuming process for me. So I appreciate the love, support, and patience of my best friend, family, and housemate, JoAnne. Additionally, the constant presence of our cats and dog served to inspire and sustain me. To Richard and Dana, my brother and sister-in-law, thank you for sharing the journey and being an important part of my story.

Finally, I share this accomplishment with my abiding source of inspiration. My mom, Jeanne W. Mattox. Her life inspired every word.

In the midst of your caregiving journey, I hope this book proves to be a blessing to you and yours. If so, I will have achieved my ultimate goal.

Contents

Summary of Chapters

Part 1—Caregiving in the Twenty-First Century 1

Chapter 1
Caregiving: Common Concern, Common Need, Common Ground 3

Caregiving is a topic of interest for everyone in the United States. It's important to understand the changing demographics in the United States and the implications for caregiving. Whether giving care or receiving care, we need to understand the process and the available resources within our community. We must be *prepared to care* if a caregiving crisis is to be avoided.

Chapter 2
How Do You Define Family? 21

The challenge of caregiving is complicated by the transformation of family systems in the United States. What constitutes a family these days? Who cares for an aging person when there is no nuclear or biological family? Who is responsible for providing care in blended families? Because there is often no obvious and/or available caregiver in a family, preplanning for care is advisable and highly recommended.

Chapter 3
Change Is the Norm: Deal with It! 33

How do families respond to the challenges of aging and illness? By understanding the basics of family systems theory, perhaps we can become a bit more tolerant and understanding of imperfect families. The reality is that all families are dysfunctional at some level. With enough stress, families will manifest some sort of dysfunction. So the goal is not perfection when it comes to caregiving. Rather, the goal is for families to meet the challenge of caregiving in effective, life-affirming ways for all involved. Families need to leverage their collective strengths, recognize the weaknesses, and seek assistance when needed (personal and professional).

Chapter 4

Caregiving Is a Family Challenge................................49

Families are delicately balanced systems. When a new "member" is introduced into the family, a new balance must be achieved. Illness and/or the challenges of aging function as destabilizing "new members" to a family system. How a family integrates the new member is dependent on the family structure, communication style, family patterns of behavior, and family beliefs.

Chapter 5

The Family Legacy of Caregiving 67

We learn so much about life by observing our families in action. This is certainly true in regard to our attitudes and approach to caregiving. It is important to recognize the legacies of caregiving that we perpetuate. Are these patterns beneficial or damaging? Obviously, we need to embrace and enhance models of caregiving that serve us well while transforming or rejecting those that don't.

Chapter 6

Long-Distance Caregiving: Bridging the Gap 81

Due to the changing nature of families and our highly mobile society, long-distance caregiving is quite common in the twenty-first century. Long-distance caregivers often experience significant expenses associated with travel, require extended time off from work, and feel guilty they cannot spend more time with the care receiver. Family disputes often arise between proximal and long-distance caregivers related to perceived disparities in caregiving responsibilities as well. Suffice it to say, long-distance caregiving requires coordination of care, proactive planning, and identification/utilization of local resources.

Chapter 7

Critter Care..95

Critters are important members of many families. As such, caregiving is a concern for aging and ill critters. Financial, emotional, and physical issues associated with the care of family critters must be discussed in order to avoid a crisis of care. This includes pet health insurance, hospice and palliative care, and guardianship issues when guardians predecease their critters.

Part 2—Assessment and Planning 111

Chapter 8
Assessment Process: Toss a SALAD! 113

Preparing to care requires the assessment of various factors. Who, what, when, where, why, and how must be assessed to develop an effective plan of care for all involved. SALAD is a mnemonic for a process that assists in assessment and planning: Schedule, Ask, Listen, Assess, and Develop. It is a recipe for creating a collaborative, compassionate, comprehensive plan of care.

Chapter 9
Goals of Care: Products of a Healthy SALAD 125

When it comes to caregiving, one size does *not* fit all. We need to understand the hopes and fears of all involved. What are the goals of care, short and long term? Is there disagreement within the family as to what is needed, desired, or required? If we fail to listen to all involved (caregivers and care receiver), we miss the opportunity to create an informed plan of care. The goals of care, which change as conditions change, serve as the guideposts to map the caregiving journey.

Chapter 10
Develop, Document, and Execute a Plan of Care: Dress the SALAD 141

When developing a plan of care, we must be aware of the available resources: personal, professional, financial, and spiritual. The integration of all available resources results in a beneficial plan of care. This is the last step in the SALAD process—develop, document, and execute the plan of care. When done well, the result is a healthy plan of care for all involved.

Chapter 11

Contrary to popular belief, hospice is not a four-letter word, nor is it something to be feared. As for palliative care, the term and concept are a mystery to most people in the United States. Hospice and palliative care are philosophies and models of care designed to serve persons with chronic and/or terminal illness in compassionate, life-giving ways. So why does the word hospice cause such angst and trepidation for patients and families? More often than not, our reactions emanate from a lack of knowledge, fear of death, denial, and avoidance. Take the first step in overcoming your fears by learning how hospice and palliative care can serve you and your family. This philosophy of care is an essential element in every plan of care.

Chapter 12

Talking with our family and friends about our final wishes is a frightening prospect for most of us. In fact, the idea is so frightening that we delay the process until there is a crisis. Having experienced and witnessed this train wreck far too many times, I want to encourage you to prepare your final gifts for those you love. It is not only about completing the needed legal forms for our health care and legal systems. Preparing for aging, illness, and ultimately death requires reflection, intention, and communication. By articulating what you want, what you need, and what is meaningful to you, your family has the necessary knowledge to care for you. What a gift!

Part 3—The Stressful Journey of Caregiving ....

Chapter 13

We must be realistic when it comes to caregiving. No matter how much we love the person, caregiving is stressful. It is important to recognize and then manage the various factors known to dramatically increase the level of stress. There are few universal truths in my world. However, one of the few is this—caregiving is stressful! And yet, most caregivers profess to be "doing *fine*." Fine? Really? When caregivers doth protest too much and proclaim to be "*fine*," I recognize the wheels are about to fall off. As caregivers, we need to recognize the signs of significant stress in ourselves and others *before* we crash. *Fine* is a fantasy. Stress is the reality for caregivers. We need to address the stress before the caregiver becomes the care receiver.

Chapter 14

Compassion Fatigue 209

Compassion fatigue is the overidentification with the suffering of another person. Professional caregivers receive training on this particular issue, but family caregivers often are unaware of the risk or the issue. Consequently, family caregivers fail to recognize the symptoms of compassion fatigue. Unaddressed, compassion fatigue compromises our ability or desire to care for another person. Caregivers describe this condition as feeling "fried" or "burned out." Knowledge of the concept and awareness of needed boundaries allow caregivers to serve others in mutually beneficial ways.

Chapter 15

Resilience: Choosing to Bounce Back 223

Resilience is an effective process of adapting well in the face of adversity. If you are resilient, you bounce back! The challenges of life may cause you to bend, but you don't break. With all the changes and subsequent transitions posed by aging and illness, the process of resilience is of great importance to caregivers and care receivers.

Part 4—The Philosophy of Collaborative Care 241

Chapter 16

May I Help You? 243

Do you have a resistance to assistance? This is an important question to ask, whether you are a caregiver or care receiver. Over the course of a long caregiving journey, we all need help from time to time.

Consequently, if you cringe at the thought of asking for or accepting help, it's important to recognize the source of resistance. Perhaps by understanding the essential nature of caregiving—interdependence—you will be better able to receive care.

Chapter 17
Tipping Points

A tipping point is the point after which everything changes. A caregiving tipping point is often the unwelcome wake-up call that requires families to respond to changing physical, cognitive, or psychosocial conditions. Caregiving tipping points often motivate families to seek additional assistance with caregiving needs as well.

Chapter 18
Flying in Formation:

If you are of the opinion that caregiving is a solo flight, I invite you to look to the skies and observe our friend the goose. Geese understand the importance of traveling together, shared leadership, encouragement during tough times, and never leaving a goose behind. Caregivers have much to learn from our friend the goose about collaborative care.

Chapter 19
Life and Loss

To live is to change. To change is to lose something or someone. To lose something or someone is to grieve. To grieve is to experience our humanity. As we companion those who are aging or ill, the repetitive process of change, loss, and transition wears on personal as well as professional caregivers. The first step in healing is recognition of the various losses. Otherwise, the losses go unnoticed and unmourned. We need to be aware of what we have to lose! Caregivers witness a tremendous amount of loss. If losses are not grieved and mourned, the losses inhibit our ability to engage life.

Chapter 20

In general, people in Western society do not understand the grief and mourning process. Grief is the internal, emotional response to loss. Mourning is the process of *doing* something with our emotions— internally and externally. It's the process of adapting to a world without the person or the thing we lost. As noted by C. S. Lewis in his classic book *A Grief Observed*, grief is frightening. So instead of confronting our grief and doing the hard work of mourning, our natural inclination is to flee. Caregivers must recognize and mourn their losses if they are to maintain good health and well-being. It is a lifelong process of touch-and-go grief and mourning.

Chapter 21

The caregiving journey often ends in the death of the person receiving care. It doesn't take a genius to predict the final act when dealing with serious or terminal illness. However, death is not something commonly or easily discussed in most households. We witness thousands of deaths via technology (television, movies, and the Internet); however, few people experience intimate death—sitting at the bedside when a loved one dies. Our absence results in ignorance of the dying process. Our ignorance causes us to fear death. Our fear of death inhibits our ability to make the necessary end-of-life plans required to live as we wish. It is paradoxical. By confronting our fears about death, we are freed to live fully.

Chapter 22

A benediction is an invocation of a blessing. It is intended to promote a sense of well-being and provide guidance. Since the journey of caregiving can be daunting, I can think of no better way to conclude our conversation than with a caregiving benediction.

Caregiving is about relationships to the past, ourselves, our families, and our friends. Jane Barton draws upon personal and professional relationships to weave insightful stories about caregiving and care receiving. Her heartfelt sharing of these stories may bring tears to your eyes. Joy and understanding. Or perhaps an "aha moment" to your soul. As a caregiver—past, present, or future—you may see yourself in some of her stories. How could Jane possibly have known what you were thinking and feeling? Well, it's quite simple. While stories are personal, caregiving is universal. The need to be in relationship with others is ubiquitous. Similar underlying themes are pervasive. Jane's masterful and humble use of stories, wherein she is willing to be vulnerable, illuminates the caregiving path. You are invited and encouraged to search your soul, to unleash your strength, and to set the wheels in motion for your own journey as a caregiver.

Understanding our core beliefs and relation to caregiving provides the foundation for planning the caregiving journey. In retrospect, as a caregiver for my mother, who lived with Alzheimer's for twenty-six years, I wish our family had better planned for caregiving rather than reacting after the axle hit the next bump in the road. If only we had known the aspects of preparing for caregiving that Jane creatively refers to as tossing the SALAD, perhaps we would have found the easier, less stressful route. However, we didn't know about SALAD back then. We never **Scheduled** a family meeting. Seldom **Asked** the important questions (especially of the care receiver). Wouldn't **Listen** to each other. Didn't have the tools to **Assess** the needs and wants of those involved. And we didn't possess the know-how to **Develop** a plan of care. In spite of ourselves, we provided loving care for our mother. There are no "do-overs" in life, nor do I want one. However, having read *Caregiving for the GENIUS*, I am prepared to do caregiving differently the next time. And, have no doubt, I *will* be a caregiver again. By planning and recognizing the relational aspects of being a caregiver, I will have a greater appreciation for the sacred journey that lies ahead. We will all be caregivers and care receivers more than once in our lives. Thus, we will have the opportunity to do caregiving differently the next time around. As Jane points out, one size (i.e., one approach) does not fit all when it comes to caregiving. In fact, one size doesn't even fit one person over two different caregiving journeys. Hence, each journey requires the creation of a new SALAD that brings together and capitalizes on the different strengths of families, friends, care receivers, and community.

There is no doubt that caregiving is highly stressful. A multitude of studies outline the dangers of caregiving: compromised health, burnout, and compassion fatigue. Jane provides hope and plants the seeds of courage that empower caregivers not only to survive the journey, but to thrive. Caregiving is not for the faint of heart. However, the journey often reveals a strong will and inner strength previously unimagined. It requires determination and resilience. Or bounce, as Jane calls it. She offers a road map to explore and to develop your own resilience that provides life-giving sustenance for the journey ahead. Resilience is the key to rebounding from the ever-present tides of change caregivers experience on a daily and sometimes hourly basis. We can each find our own gifts for rebounding in the face of adversity by using our knowledge, courage, and relationships as a springboard. There isn't a laundry list of steps or a perfect recipe to create an attitude of resilience. Instead, you will need to reach deep within and without to shape your own attitudes and become resilient. I encourage you to take up Jane's challenge to find your bounce. Shape your attitude. And strengthen your resilience. It will serve you well in navigating the myriad of changes well beyond the caregiver journey.

Jane has come to the table with gifts of wisdom and knowledge for you to consider and share with family and friends. Once done, you will be well prepared to find your own truths and to define your own caregiving path. I imagine many readers, like myself, will subsequently find the courage to understand and embrace the changes brought on by caregiving and care receiving. Many thanks to Jane for gracefully sharing her stories that reflect the common experience of caregiving. For sharing her soul with our souls. And for challenging us to choose our attitudes, to reach out to others, and to design our unique paths as caregivers.

Cheryl A. Siefert, Master of Nonprofit Management
Executive Director
Parkinson Association of the Rockies

Caregiving for the GENIUS specifically invites and encourages Boomers (those persons born between 1946 and 1964) to prepare to care—to intentionally plan for the experience of caregiving and care receiving. Boomers are changing the demographics in the United States in significant and somewhat frightening ways. It is hard to ignore seventy-eight million people requiring ever-increasing levels of care related to chronic illness and advancing age. Every day, ten thousand Boomers turn sixty-five years of age. Every day, countless people feel overwhelmed by the daunting challenges posed by aging, illness, and associated disabilities.

This Boomer age wave is a societal, family, and individual challenge. Whether a Boomer, a parent of a Boomer, a child of a Boomer, or a professional serving Boomers, you will be impacted by this wave of aging Boomers. So I invite you to consider your specific situation carefully. Prepare to care before the age wave hits your shores. And if the waves are lapping at your front door, do not despair! Your sneakers may initially get soggy, but there is dry land in your future. Take a deep breath. Read this book. And take one step at a time. There is hope if you choose to be proactive in planning for care.

Although we are an age-denying society, we must face the reality of our situation. We *are* getting older! If we are to have any chance at aging well (whatever that means to you), we must be proactive. We *must* anticipate needs, identify resources, and establish our goals of care (personal preferences). You need not be a Boomer to benefit from this book. Caregiving is a universal, timeless concern. So, Boomer or not, keep reading! There is something here for everyone.

The issue of caregiving is a common concern in the United States and, consequently, a common cause. *Caregiving for the GENIUS* serves to explore the essential aspects of caregiving and care receiving. I have witnessed far too many families that were dazed and confused when caregiving needs arose or escalated. The experience of caregiving is not easy; however, it need not be devastating or debilitating for families. The mantra of "prepare to care" compels families to have the needed conversations. Ask the questions. Explore the options. Consider the various scenarios. Imagine "what if." We are not clairvoyant. We can't accurately predict the future. However, we need to consider the realistic possibilities and plan accordingly.

Preplanning for life is not a novel approach or idea. We are encouraged to preplan other aspects of our lives: finances, final arrangements, career tracks, and taxes. So why not caregiving? One thing for sure, by investing your time, talents, and treasures in a plan of care, you will look like a GENIUS when caregiving becomes a concern for you and your family. However, I am realistic about the option to preplan; few people preplan much of anything. We wait until something happens, and then we *react* to the crisis. As we all know from experience, we don't make the best decisions when the fur is flying and emotions are raw. We are much better served if we have a plan in place that outlines a general approach to and philosophy of caregiving. Considering in advance the who, what, when, where, why, and how of caregiving and care receiving alleviates stress and mitigates fear for the entire family.

Life does not follow a preordained script. Life deviates from the norm unexpectedly. However, we do know with certainty that every person will age (physically and cognitively) and therefore be at increased risk of chronic and/or terminal illness. Based on that certainty, it is important to develop a preferred plan of care. We can't accurately predict the details of our physical or cognitive demise. However, we can reflect on what constitutes an acceptable quality of life. What aspects of your life are essential? What aspects are optional? Where is your line in the sand? Your philosophy of life will serve to guide those in charge of your care when you are no longer able to articulate your wishes. A gift indeed!

Caregiving for the GENIUS addresses aspects of care often omitted— evolution of care; the need to preplan for care; attitudes, beliefs, and legacies of care. The majority of caregiving books on the market today focus on the logistics of caregiving and specific resources. Granted, this is important. However, the first step in developing a plan of care is to realize how we *feel* about caregiving and care receiving and how those feelings inform the decisions we make. What family, cultural, and spiritual norms inform your decisions? How did you learn to care for others? Do you easily accept help? These types of questions require self-reflection and self-knowledge.

Caregiving is more than a logistical issue to be solved and endured. Caregiving engages your entire being—mind, body, and spirit.

I opted to focus on the emotional, spiritual, and relational aspects of caring. What does it feel like to give and receive care? What are the burdens as well as the blessings inherent in caregiving? How can we engage the journey of caregiving in life-giving ways for all concerned? Although I am writing *Caregiving for the GENIUS*, I do not profess to know all things related to caregiving! Instead, I humbly offer the lessons learned through my personal and professional experiences as a caregiver.

As I considered writing this book, I realized that I have been preparing my entire life to write *this* book. Not because I believe myself to be *the* expert on caregiving. But, instead, I wrote the book because I have something meaningful to say about the experience of caregiving and care receiving. The essence of my message is rooted in experiences, education, and encounters with amazing people over the past fifty-six years. It is truly my delight (and at times my challenge!) to weave the various threads of my life into what I hope will be a beneficial story for other caregivers and care receivers.

My best teachers and mentors were those people I served—my family, friends, and hospice patients. The lived experience reveals the heart and soul of caregiving. The stories. So I offer my story and the stories of others to inspire, to inform, and to console people in similar situations. My interactions with individuals inspired all the stories; however, the characters in the stories are often composite figures. Names, locations, and situational details have been changed to honor the confidentiality of all persons, with the exception of my immediate family members. I have no doubt that my parents and my godparents (all of whom are deceased) would allow me full disclosure for the greater good. If, by chance, I have incorrectly assessed their wishes, they can express their displeasure with me at a later date, *much* later! That is a risk I am willing to take. I cannot speak to the issue of caregiving without referring to my foundational, formative caregiving experiences within my family.

I have to admit, I feel a bit "exposed" and vulnerable sharing some of my stories. But, over the past ten years, I have realized that vulnerability ignites the senses. I feel most alive when vulnerable and raw. As a dear friend of mine says, "I am living life to the tips of my hairs!" Also, vulnerability breeds vulnerability. As I "go deep" in sharing my story, you are invited to "go deep" and reflect on your situation. Caregiving can be a daunting, challenging journey. It is not only a logistical issue; it is intensely emotional and spiritual. If my stories serve to inform, inspire, and guide you—fabulous! My fervent hope is that you find something of benefit between the covers of this book.

Caregiving begins and ends with listening. To care for others and to care for ourselves, we must listen well. My mom is the person who taught me the art of listening and embodied the role of caregiver. My apprenticeship began at the age of three. Every morning, Mom and I visited neighbors who needed nothing more than someone who cared! Mom and I sat around the kitchen tables of our neighbors sipping hot tea, sharing stories, and listening. Mom rarely said anything. Instead, she honored the person before her by being present to their joys and sorrows. She listened to their hopes and their fears. She resisted the temptation to "fix" or judge people. Instead, she allowed them the safe space to give voice to their lives, the good and the bad.

When my mom died in 1981, countless people reflected on the gift of listening that my mom had graciously given them throughout her life. They said, "Your mom always made me feel like the most important person in the world. I knew if I came to your mom, she would hear me. She would listen. Your mom helped me more than I can ever say. She changed my life." Listening. Transformational? Memorable? Absolutely! As caregivers (personal and professional alike), we serve well when we choose to listen first. Compassionate, competent care emanates from a foundational understanding and appreciation of the person. Having learned at the feet of my mom, I am mindful to approach family, friends, and clients with open ears, open arms, an open mind, and an open and accepting heart. To care well for others requires our entire being. A high calling indeed.

By describing the experience of caregiving from the inside out—exploring how caregiving *feels* and affects individuals and families—the impetus for planning becomes obvious. If we fail to plan well, we will suffer the consequences—physically, financially, emotionally, relationally, and spiritually. *Caregiving for the GENIUS* provides the information, the insights, and the inspiration for Boomers (and others) to develop a plan of care—to prepare to care from the inside out.

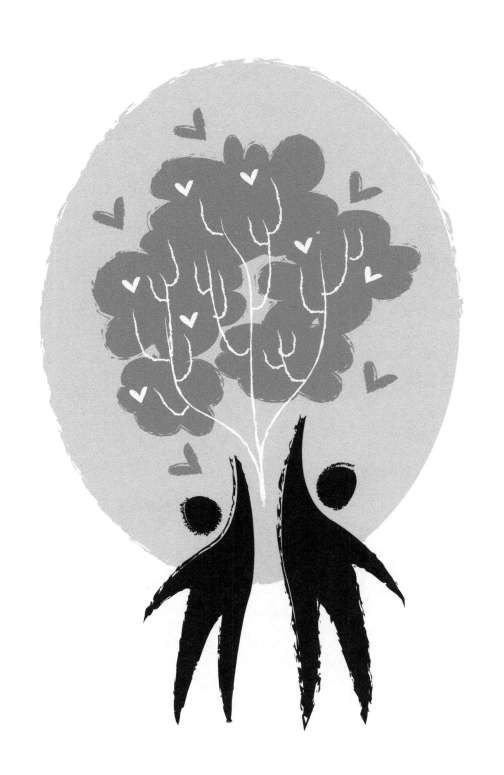

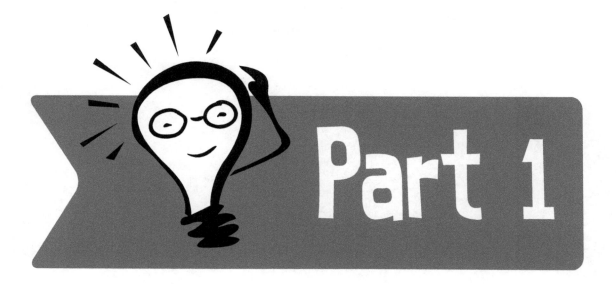

Caregiving in the Twenty-First Century

Let's begin by exploring the state of the union related to caregiving. Pick up a newspaper or glance at the Internet. Caregiving is obviously a hot topic today. We'll examine the demographic trends and societal changes in the United States fueling the growing concerns related to caregiving. We'll also discuss the destabilizing nature of aging and illness. If you are diagnosed with a chronic or terminal illness, the challenge is personal. However, the impact of your diagnosis is systemic. Everyone who knows you is affected by your compromised physical and/or cognitive condition. We'll also consider the family legacy of caregiving. Some legacies are worthy of continuation, while others are ripe for transformation. The common issue of long-distance caregiving necessitates modifications to traditional models of care. Finally, we'll chat about a topic near and dear to my heart, critter care. The four-legged, furry members of your family require a plan of care as well.

Chapter 1

Caregiving: Common Concern, Common Need, Common Ground

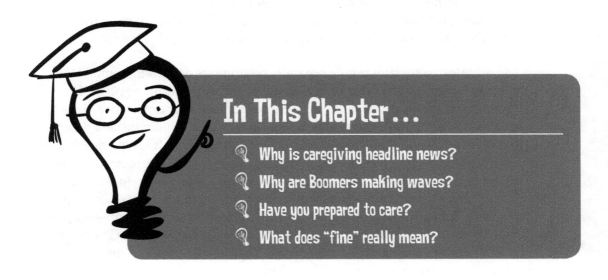

In This Chapter...

- 💡 Why is caregiving headline news?
- 💡 Why are Boomers making waves?
- 💡 Have you prepared to care?
- 💡 What does "fine" really mean?

Caregiving is a universal concern. Young and old. Male and female. Rich and poor. Educated and illiterate. All races. All ethnicities. All beliefs. Caregiving is not discriminating. Over the course of a lifetime, we will *all* be called to care for someone we know (family or friend). Furthermore, we will *all* be care recipients as we decline physically and cognitively due to aging and/or illness. Caregiving is thus a common concern and common need worthy of our collective attention. Common ground—a good place to begin a productive conversation!

In the United States, an unprecedented demographic shift (the Boomer generation) has resulted in an age wave of epic proportions, sometimes referred to as the Silver Tsunami. According to the US Census Bureau in December 2012, the population aged sixty-five and older will more than double between 2012 and 2060 (from forty-three million to ninety-two million people). Additionally, the greatest increase will be seen in the "oldest of the old," those persons aged eighty-five and older (six million to eighteen million persons). Currently, one in seven persons is over the age of sixty-five. By 2060, that ratio will be one in five persons. So the growth in our senior population far exceeds that of younger generations. The repercussions of increased longevity, chronic illness, escalating costs of health care, and alternative family structures challenge aging Boomers and their families at every turn. We must understand the societal changes if we are to anticipate and meet the caregiving needs of our aging population. Knowledge is power. Knowledge enables us to be proactive instead of reactive. To meet the challenges of caregiving, we need to know what we are up against.

In addition to societal trends, we must be students of human nature. How do we typically respond to the challenges (and opportunities) posed by aging and illness? What influences our responses? Past experience? Fear? Faith? Facts? Denial? The reality is this—few people anticipate caregiving needs and subsequently prepare to care. Instead, we wait for "something" to happen—a tipping point—that necessitates a response. Furthermore, even when chaos reigns, we will calmly assure those wanting to help that we are fine. *Fine*. Really? How do you define fine? Our resistance to ask for help and receive help is *the* biggest barrier to improving the journey of caregiving for all involved. So we need to identify our source(s) of resistance. Caregiving need not be a solitary, isolating journey. Sharing the journey with others transforms the experience in life-giving ways.

The Call to Care

I am—by nature, nurture, and necessity—a caregiver. I have cared for my parents, godparents, and friends who were challenged by aging and illness. As a hospice chaplain, palliative care educator, spiritual director, and educational consultant, I serve as a professional caregiver. I have also been a care receiver at times over the course of my fifty-six-year journey. Since you are reading this book, I imagine we share some common experiences. Perhaps you are a fellow Boomer who is caring for a spouse, partner, friend, sibling, parent, or child. Maybe you are a caregiver by profession. Or maybe, just maybe, you are beginning to wonder who will care for you—now or in the future. Regardless of your caregiving situation, the journey can be daunting in the twenty-first century for a variety of reasons, reasons we will discuss momentarily.

As an educator, I want to ensure that we are all on the same page when I use the term "caregiver." For the purposes of this book, *caregiver* refers to a person who provides unpaid care to a family member (human or critter) or friend. The person may or may not be trained to serve in this role. You may hear the term "informal caregiver." Means the same thing. In contrast, a *professional caregiver* is compensated for the professional care provided (medical, psychological, pastoral, etc.).

I am a firm believer that knowledge is power. If we are to age well, we need to understand the process of aging. Fundamentally, aging is a continuous process of change and transition complicated by illness and associated disabilities.

Few people will complete the journey of life without needing assistance from family members and health care professionals. So we'll all be called to care for our loved ones, and we'll all need care. Best we engage the journey with our eyes wide open!

Just the Facts

We live in extraordinary times, don't we? In the United States over the past century, we have seen advances in medical technology, pharmaceutical discoveries, and improvements in hygiene that have significantly increased life expectancies. Over the course of the twentieth century, we witnessed an increase in life expectancy of over thirty years. Unprecedented! The Social Security Administration has an online calculator that estimates your life expectancy based on your current age and gender. Since I am currently fifty-six years old and female, I am estimated to live to the venerable age of 85.7 years. My male counterpart is expected to live until 82.8 years. Sorry guys, women still reign supreme when it comes to longevity!

Now, I am all about enjoying a longer life. However, with increased longevity comes the challenge of maintaining and managing our health. The only way we will *enjoy* a longer life is to engage the journey with our eyes wide open. Few of us will complete the journey without some bumps and bruises along the way. The Centers for Disease Control and Prevention reported in 2011 that 80 percent of older persons (age sixty-five and older) have at least one chronic condition, while 50 percent have at least two chronic conditions. The reality is this—the carrot and the stick. There is the hope of a longer life. However, advanced age will require ever-increasing levels of care for most of us.

Over the past decade, various foundations and organizations conducted caregiver surveys. The results highlight the tremendous responsibility assumed by family and friends for those challenged by aging, illness, and disability. I don't want to bore you with a lot of data and statistics. But a foundational understanding of the situation is necessary to instill a sense of urgency, an urgency to develop personal and systemic plans of care for our aging population. According to the Family Caregiver Alliance in November 2012, in the United States, it is estimated that:

- approximately sixty-six million people serve as caregivers;

- a majority of caregivers (86 percent) care for a relative;

- caregivers provide on average 20.4 hours of care per week;

- the value of the care provided is $450 billion annually;

- 61 percent of all caregivers are employed;

- the typical caregiver is a forty-eight-year-old female;

- the typical care receiver is a seventy-five-year-old female;

- 66 percent of caregivers are women; 34 percent are men;

- the average duration of the caregiving journey is 4.6 years;

- the majority of care receivers rely *solely* on one person for care.

Caregiving statistics are updated annually by organizations such as AARP, Family Caregiver Alliance, Alzheimer's Association, and MetLife Mature Market Institute. Numbers may vary between reports depending on the source of the data. As you might imagine, it is difficult to gather the caregiving data from family caregivers. However, all reports conclude that caregiving is a tremendous societal challenge that is projected to increase in magnitude with the aging of the Boomer generation.

Who Is Called to Care?

Do I have your attention? The numbers are concerning, to say the very least. If you thought you would fly under the radar screen, I am your wake-up call! We will all be called to care. We will all need care. And we will *all* require more care than we ever imagined due to the previously noted demographic trends. Increasing life expectancy. Higher incidence of chronic illness. Increased levels of required care. Astronomical health care costs. Disproportionate numbers of caregivers versus care receivers. These are determining factors in how we will age. Instead of merely hoping for the best, let's work to ensure that our increased longevity proves to be a blessing rather than a curse.

We also need to recognize how we typically respond to the call for care. In Western society, when called, we have a tendency to assume the role of primary caregiver, a person who assumes the lion's share of responsibility for care. Sometimes we do this out of necessity—there is no one else available. But quite often we opt to be the primary caregiver due to cultural or family norms, a sense of duty, family expectations, pride, inability to ask for help, or desire for control.

If you are a primary caregiver, I am not disparaging your approach to care. However, I will caution you. Because the nature of caregiving has changed dramatically over the past fifty to one hundred years, the journey of caregiving is longer, harder, and more complicated. If you choose to engage the role of caregiver alone, you are at high risk of compromising your own health and sense of well-being. What happens if you have your own health care crisis, predecease your loved one, or decide you've had enough? Who will then assume the role of caregiver? These are critically important questions to address for the caregiver and care receiver. **Part 4** offers information about communal approaches to caregiving, an approach that allows others to share in the responsibilities of care as well as the blessings. It is pretty much a given that we will all be called to care for a family member or friend. However, we need not fly solo.

How Were You Called to Care?

The manner in which we are called to care informs our experience of caregiving as well. Did you get "the call" at 3:00 a.m. about your dad's stroke? Or perhaps you have been preparing to care for your mother who was diagnosed with Alzheimer's disease five years ago. Whether the call is sudden or anticipated, this detour in your life is disruptive, right? This is not what you had planned. Consequently, you may feel frustrated, angry, scared, sad, and conflicted. Rest assured, your reaction is normal. However, the call to care requires a course correction. Initially, you may feel like an alien in a foreign land. However, step by step, the path unfolds in amazing ways, revealing not only challenges but also opportunities along the way.

The Changing Nature of Care

Due to the increase in life expectancy, the call to care has changed dramatically just in my lifetime. Caregiving is not a short-term proposition anymore. The average duration of care is 4.6 years. Please note, the duration of care will increase dramatically in the next thirty years as the Boomer generation ages. As noted previously, chronic illness is the norm, not the exception. Many chronic conditions persist for decades, requiring additional care as the illness progresses. Additionally, the greatest risk of developing dementia is advanced age.

Dementia is not a specific disease. Rather, it is an overarching term that includes a variety of diseases and conditions. Dementia occurs when brain cells die or malfunction, resulting in cognitive impairment. Memory loss, speech impairment, lack of recognition, impaired motor skills, and inability to think abstractly are symptoms of dementia. Additionally, the cognitive impairment must be significant enough to interfere with daily life.

Alzheimer's disease is the most common type of dementia in the United States. It is also known to be the most arduous caregiving journey due to the

Houston, We Have a Problem!

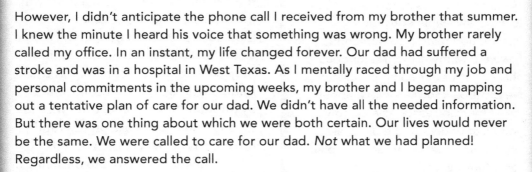

In 1992, I worked as an exploration geologist for a major oil company in Oklahoma City. Unexpectedly, our entire office was transferred to Houston, Texas. My transfer was merely one of many major life changes that year. Within a span of nine months, I got divorced, moved, and changed jobs. By midyear, I felt like Chicken Little! In fact, I kept a hard hat on my desk just in case something else threatened to fall out of the sky!

However, I didn't anticipate the phone call I received from my brother that summer. I knew the minute I heard his voice that something was wrong. My brother rarely called my office. In an instant, my life changed forever. Our dad had suffered a stroke and was in a hospital in West Texas. As I mentally raced through my job and personal commitments in the upcoming weeks, my brother and I began mapping out a tentative plan of care for our dad. We didn't have all the needed information. But there was one thing about which we were both certain. Our lives would never be the same. We were called to care for our dad. *Not* what we had planned! Regardless, we answered the call.

I used the nine hours on the road to consider my fate—and to rage! My focus bounced between a myriad of concerns. I felt as if I were in an emotional blender— one minute feeling hopeful, the next despairing. I even considered going AWOL. I didn't know if I could handle one more big change in my life. But as I continued to drive, I recognized the highway as a metaphor of my life. Yes, I had encountered many detours in the past year that changed the course of my life. There were times when I felt as if I were four-wheeling in the wilderness! And yet, my off-road experience proved to be a blessing in so many ways. I visited places unimagined, glorious places. Met amazing people. Expanded my worldview. Recharged my weary spirit. And reclaimed my passion for life. Hmm. I realized in that moment that I had a choice to make. I could view this moment as life limiting *or* life expanding. I could remain angry and lament the loss of *my* plans and become embittered. Or I could once again be fascinated by a detour and shift into four-wheel drive. Since I haven't seen smooth pavement in the subsequent twenty-one years, I am forever grateful that I chose to be fascinated.

We Must Understand the Journey of Alzheimer's Disease

I encourage you to visit the Alzheimer's Association website (alz.org) to download the annual *Facts and Figures* report as well as other available educational information related to dementia. If we are to meet the tremendous challenges of our aging population, we *must* be knowledgeable about Alzheimer's disease. As a caregiver, you must understand the disease process in order to proactively plan for future needs.

IMPORTANT!

duration and intensity of care required. The Alzheimer's Association publishes *Facts and Figures* every year. Included in the report is disease-specific information and updated statistics about the prevalence and mortality rates.

Currently, there are 5.2 million people estimated to have Alzheimer's disease in the United States. There are 15.4 million people (family and friends) providing the needed care to those persons with the disease. By 2050, it is estimated that fourteen million people will suffer from the disease. You do the math. The projected amount of care required is mind boggling. Families confronted by this daunting challenge are wise to understand the disease process and proactively develop a plan of care. Of all the challenges related to the aging of the Boomer generation, the escalating incidence of Alzheimer's disease is the most frightening. Individuals, families, communities, and health care systems will be pushed to the limit (possibly beyond) as we attempt to meet the demand for dementia-specific care.

Increased Expectations of Care

So much has changed since I served as a caregiver to my mom over forty years ago. One of the most significant changes is the level of responsibility that families must now assume when loved ones are discharged from the hospital. For example, after my mom was diagnosed with breast cancer, she had a unilateral mastectomy. My mom remained in the hospital for three to four days following the surgery. Today, it is not uncommon for a unilateral mastectomy to be done on an outpatient or overnight basis. As a result, families are expected to provide higher levels of care—care they may not feel comfortable or qualified to provide.

The Need to Be Known

I experienced one of the most devastating aspects of dementia when caring for my godmother, Aunt Jane. It is shocking when someone you loved your entire life no longer recognizes you. For those families dealing with a progressive dementia such as Alzheimer's disease, this is the harsh reality. There will come a time when the person you care for no longer knows you. Personally, I don't believe you can prepare yourself adequately for that moment. It will be devastating. It will be emotional. And you will grieve mightily. Be gentle with yourself, and get the support you need to continue the journey. One step at a time.

Example

Several years ago, I witnessed the consequences of shorter hospital stays on family members. I was sitting in the surgical waiting room of a hospital. A friend of mine was there for a simple outpatient procedure, and I was her ride. Surgical waiting rooms are interesting, aren't they? You witness a myriad of emotions as tragic and miraculous news is shared with family and friends. You try to respect the privacy of others, but it is impossible not to overhear many of the conversations. As I sat waiting, I noticed a woman sitting by herself and looking incredibly anxious. My heart went out to her as I wondered what her particular situation might be. I didn't have to wonder very long.

A surgeon entered the room and made a beeline for this woman. In short order, he shared the news about her husband. He evidently had shoulder surgery to reattach a tendon. All went well, according to the surgeon. However, he did share that the damage to the shoulder was more extensive than originally thought. Consequently, the recovery would take at least six weeks. Additionally, he cautioned that the arm could not be lowered below the level of the shoulder. Imagine holding your arm over your head for six weeks! Furthermore, there was *not* a brace to ensure the arm would remain elevated. He then told the woman that her husband would be discharged the next day after a brief consultation with a physical therapist. With that, the surgeon did an about face and headed for the exit.

The woman had the presence of mind to grab the surgeon's shirt and pull him back. She had some questions and concerns! The surgeon looked a bit

Ignorance Is *Not* Bliss!

As Sarah drove her mom home from the hospital, she reflected on the events of the past twelve hours. So much had happened in a short period of time. Earlier today, she and her mom arrived at the hospital for an outpatient surgery, a unilateral mastectomy. Sarah thought she was well prepared for the day; however, this evening she felt totally overwhelmed! When she looked over at the figure of her mother, dozing peacefully in the front seat, her heart ached. She had never seen her mother this vulnerable. Sarah had never felt so needed. Although she wanted to help her mother, Sarah was beginning to realize the implications of her mother's illness. As a result, Sarah was feeling incredibly anxious.

Based on her conversations with the surgeon following the operation, it was obvious that her mother had been protecting Sarah for the past few weeks—protecting her from the truth of the prognosis. Now, Sarah felt ill prepared for the path that was unfolding. This morning, Sarah was a daughter driving her mom to the hospital. Tonight, she is a CNA, nurse, physical therapist, pharmacist, counselor, chaplain, insurance specialist, cook, laundress, maid, and parent to her mother! These new roles are in addition to the roles she has within her own family—married with three children. Oh, and let's not forget the sixty- to eighty-hour-a-week job that serves to support her family! Is it any wonder that Sarah is feeling overwhelmed?

This scenario is quite common due to changes within our health care system. The good news is that some hospitals are working to improve the discharge process, better preparing families for the transition from hospital to home. However, we can learn a lesson from Sarah's story. Be proactive as a family caregiver. Prior to surgical procedures, gather the needed information to develop a plan of care. Who, what, when, where, why, how, and for how long? Your inquisitiveness will serve you well.

miffed, but he had little choice. This woman was not about to be ignored or dismissed. The woman then began explaining the reality of her situation. She and her husband lived in a rural area of the state on a ranch. The nearest neighbor was fifty miles down the road. They had no children. She planned to be the primary caregiver for her husband based on the surgeon's initial assessment. Now, instead of a two-week recovery, they were looking at six weeks, with the complicating factor of immobility. The problem with that—she had a full-time job that required a three-hour commute each day. Furthermore, her husband was right handed. Guess what? He was now required to keep his right hand waving in the air for six weeks. How did the surgeon envision her husband getting through the day without significant help? What would he suggest she do to adequately care for her husband?

The surgeon looked nonplussed. Shrugged his shoulders. And then said, "Well, I guess you better get some help." With that, he left the room! Really? Seriously? I could not believe my ears. Having companioned my parents through many surgeries, I dealt with some rather callous, abrasive surgeons. But this particular doctor was exceptionally arrogant and dismissive. He embodied the disconnect too often experienced by patients and their families. Doctors prescribe a plan of care and disconnect from *how* that plan will be implemented. The "hows" of implementing a plan of care are critically important. But the reality is that families are too often left to figure out the "hows" on their own. Trial by fire.

As a society, as families, and as individuals, we are challenged by the implications of increased life expectancy, increased incidence of chronic illness, and inadequate health care systems. The onus is on us to prepare to care. We must be advocates and champions for ourselves and for our families. So as not to become complacent or haughty, acknowledge that the unexpected will rise up to surprise and confound you—just like the woman in the surgical waiting room. Preparing to care requires flexibility and resilience. If our initial plan of care proves inadequate, we must bounce back with Plan B. We will discuss the important process of resilience in **Chapter 15**.

Boomers Are Making Waves

Based on the demographics noted previously, Boomers are, and will continue to be, important players in the caregiving journey. Today, I can almost guarantee that a Boomer is part of every caregiving conversation and journey. Whether a caregiver, care receiver, friend, child, sibling, or parent, the Boomer has a voice in the caregiving journey. Hence, we are well advised to know some general attitudes, tendencies, and expectations of this generation.

Generational Characteristics

Boomers, those of us born between 1946 and 1964, are an interesting breed of cat, eh? We attract attention by our mere size if nothing else, an estimated seventy-eight million people. Every day, ten thousand Boomers turn sixty-five years old. If you are in the business of serving seniors, this statistic is music to your ears. You don't have to worry about demand for your services. Instead, as a service provider, your challenge is meeting the demand for services. Additionally, you have the challenge of satisfying a very demanding generation.

When dealing with issues of aging, illness, and disability, I can almost guarantee you that a Boomer will be involved in the discussion. Due to the significant size of the Boomer generation, there are a lot of us running around! Additionally, our age range puts us right in the middle of the caregiving issue, hence the designation as the "sandwich" generation. Many Boomers are companioning their aging parents while also dealing with their own aging process. The squeeze is felt by Boomers with children who have yet to reach adulthood or resist leaving the nest. The squeeze is quite severe for families with children who have physical, cognitive, or behavioral disabilities. So Boomers know the trinity of caregiving all too well—care of parents, care of self and contemporaries, and care of children. Consequently, to understand the current challenges and opportunities related to caregiving, we *must* understand the characteristics of the Boomer generation: attitudes, expectations, beliefs, values, and lifestyles.

I am usually hesitant to make assumptions about large groups of people. Stereotypes limit, if not derail, our interactions with other people. However, I think it is beneficial to have a basis of understanding from which to work. From this foundational knowledge, we can then seek to understand the individual. So, as you read the list of traits associated with the Boomer generation, please do not be offended. You will not agree with all the characteristics noted. However, it is important to recognize the general tendencies and attitudes of the generation to appreciate our reactions to the challenges posed by aging and illness. Our expectations, our hopes, our fears, and our beliefs affect our responses to life. Recognizing the roots of our reactions related to caregiving results in efficient, beneficial course corrections. With that said, the Boomer generation is characterized in the following ways:

- Resistant to the aging process
- Better educated than our parents
- Workaholics
- Enthusiastic consumers of material goods
- Egocentric
- Demanding of extraordinary service
- Impatient
- Health and fitness conscious
- Extravagant
- Commonly divorced
- Independent, individualistic
- Skeptical of authority
- Self-reflective
- Goal oriented
- Competitive
- Optimistic
- Effective communicators
- Spiritual, not necessarily religious
- Mobile

Implications for Caregiving and Care Receiving

In subsequent chapters, we will address how the generational tendencies of Boomers impact the experience of caregiving and care receiving. Understanding how Boomers "see" the world provides a basis for compassionate, collaborative communication. For example, knowing that Boomers are an age-denying generation, is it any wonder that we fail to proactively plan for our ultimate demise? We prefer to discuss the options around Botox treatments, plastic surgery, and other age-defying treatments. Ultimately, our fears related to aging and death cause most of us to procrastinate—to live as if we are immortal! Too often we recognize the reality of our mortality in the midst of the crisis—the devastating moment when we begin lamenting our lack of preparation and planning.

In **Chapter 2**, we will discuss the implications of the shrinking family and alternative lifestyles for aging Boomers. With fewer children to care for aging parents, who will be called to care? Unlike our parents, Boomers typically have not been frugal. Even the Boomers who deviated from the norm and chose to invest for retirement were negatively impacted by the market collapse in 2008. So, if we don't have large nuclear families to companion us as we age, how will we afford all the care that we need?

As we address these and many other questions, reflect on the traits and attitudes of Boomers. It will all become clear and the light will dawn! There are reasons why many Boomers (and others) have not planned for the likelihood of increased care due to aging and illness. I am not making excuses for Boomers, or for anyone else, who fail (failed) to anticipate future caregiving needs. Rather, I seek to understand the "whys" behind the resistance. We must identify the points of resistance to know how to invite and to encourage Boomers to proactively plan. *Telling* people what to do is rarely effective, particularly with Boomers. Remember, we question authority!

Consequently, in subsequent chapters, I will resist telling you what to do. Instead, I invite you to consider a different way of engaging the journey of caregiving, whether caregiver or care receiver. Be proactive instead of reactive. Be fascinated instead of frightened. Know instead of wonder.

Preparing to care requires more than a list of service providers and community resources. We must prepare to care from the inside out—know thyself and seek to know those you serve.

Don't Wait for the Crisis

When I first began working as a palliative care educator many years ago, one of my first projects was to create a program on caregiving. My mission was to develop a training program for caregivers. Although I was inexperienced in the field of hospice and palliative care, I knew the journey of caregiving from personal experience. Consequently, I was passionate about creating a beneficial program for caregivers and care receivers. Based on my own experience, I wanted to convince families that preplanning for care was essential for all concerned. Why wait for a crisis?

After months of research and review of existing programs, I developed what I thought was an irresistible curriculum for caregivers. What I failed to realize initially was that regardless of the worthiness of the training, caregivers did not have the time, the inclination, or the energy to attend a workshop or class! Caregivers were too busy caring for their loved ones. Well, duh? Now what?

Well, if caregivers (personal) did not have time to attend a class, perhaps professional caregivers would be interested in learning about innovative approaches to caregiving. They in turn could then become advocates within the community and encourage their clients and families to prepare to care. This proved to be a much better, successful approach to caregiver training.

Based on attendance, evaluations, and personal testimonials, the caregiving workshops were successful events. However, I remained disappointed because the majority of families I met at the workshops waited until a caregiving crisis arose to develop a plan of care. Granted, some families were blindsided by an accident, unexpected medical crisis, or tragedy. However, for families that had a diagnosis of Alzheimer's disease, MS, cancer, or some other progressive illness, why were they hesitant to prepare to care? Why were they reluctant to ask other family members and friends for the help they needed?

To determine the underlying reason(s) for this observed procrastination and reluctance to ask for help, I held focus groups with caregivers and care receivers. I worked with a friend who is an expert in the design and facilitation of focus groups. The discussions were insightful and thought provoking. Upon reflection, some obvious themes emerged from the focus groups. People often waited until the wheels fell off because of:

- denial;
- pride;
- fear of rejection;
- lack of information about the disease process;
- cultural and family norms;
- privacy/secrecy;
- control;
- isolation.

In most instances, a tipping point is required to prompt a primary caregiver to ask for help or to rethink the current plan of care (if one even existed). The tipping point is a game changer in the disease process that prompts an increase in care or a different kind of care. For many caregivers, incontinence is the tipping point. This prompts discussions about transitioning to long-term care communities or contracting with home health services. Obviously, each caregiving journey is unique and dependent on the individuals involved. Therefore, the tipping point will vary from family to family. Caregivers have a mental "line in the sand." So I invite you to discuss your "line in the sand" with your care receiver, other family members, and friends. You need not wait to be pushed across the line before considering viable options of care. Avoid the crisis by courageously planning for future needs. Being proactive will serve you well.

Fine Is Usually *Not* Fine

I am always amazed by our customary response to the question "How are you?" More than likely when asked, you respond with "Fine!" What is fascinating about the response is that you claim to be fine despite the fact you were just laid off. You can't pay your mortgage. Your dog ran away. Your son wrecked your car. And you are the sole caregiver for your mother with Alzheimer's disease and have been for the past five years. But, hey, you are *fine*! I can't tell you how many times I have used the same response to deflect the inquiries of others and remain in my reassuring state of denial. To admit that I am *not* fine would be to recognize the reality of my situation. I would also have to acknowledge that perhaps I need and want help. Those of us who are products of Western society find it very difficult to admit we need help. We were raised to be independent, self-reliant, autonomous, and in control. Asking for help goes against the grain. We bristle at the insinuation that we are inadequate or incapable of meeting the challenge.

Historically, my typical approach to caregiving has been the Lone Ranger model. I heard the call to care. I hopped on my trusty steed and charged ahead (usually without a clue as to where I was going). Believing that I could do all things (because that was how I was raised), I initially resisted the advice and help of others. Instead, I sat tall in the saddle, smiling in the face of adversity. Regardless of the caregiving challenge, I was arrogant enough to think I could actually do it all by myself. Silly me! I may not be Mensa material, but I am a quick study. Since my first experience of caregiving at the young age of fifteen, I have learned that I cannot be all things to all people. It is okay to ask for help. In fact, people are honored to be asked! And "*fine*" is a *Red Flag Warning*. The train is headed downhill, the brakes have failed, and a crash is imminent. In other words, *take cover*!

Red Flag Warning

A Red Flag Warning is a warning issued by the US National Weather Service when conditions are ripe for wildfires. Being from Colorado, I am all too aware of the danger posed by drought conditions and the subsequent threat of wildfires. In regard to caregiving, there are also warning signs of imminent danger and destruction that need to be recognized and heeded if we are to avoid a disaster.

Definition

In **Chapter 16**, we will explore in more detail our resistance to asking for and receiving help. We need to be sensitive to cultural expectations related to caregiving as well as family norms. Once again, instead of telling others how to engage the journey, we invite people to consider different models of care. There is more than one way to companion those needing care. Just remember, in all instances, *fine* is usually *not* fine!

To Summarize...

- Caregiving is a common concern, a common need, and the common ground on which we stand. If we are to compassionately and competently meet the needs of our aging population, we must be proactive instead of reactive.

- The demographic shift caused by the aging of the Boomer generation is straining our health care systems, long-term care services, and family systems. Boomers are central to the discussion of caregiving since they currently serve as dual caregivers (aging parents and maturing children) as well as being recipients of care.

- If you have not seriously considered how you will care for your aging or ill family members, you should. Furthermore, who will care for you as you age or are challenged by illness? There is no need to wait for a crisis to develop a plan of action! Proaction trumps reaction every time. Be brave. Be bold. Prepare to care!

- Remember that "*fine*" is a four-letter word when it comes to caregiving! When you or others adamantly claim to be doing *fine*, perhaps Shakespeare has the correct assessment of the situation. "Methinks thou dost protest too much." *Fine* is a Red Flag Warning. Pay attention and explore options for needed assistance.

Chapter 2

How Do You Define Family?

In This Chapter...

- Who is your family?
- Who will care for you?
- Do we expect too much of families?

Today, I am hard pressed to offer a concise and accurate definition of "family." There is no *traditional* family in the United States. Our family units come in all shapes and sizes. There are many reasons for the evolution of the family system, but Boomers are responsible for many of the changes witnessed over the past fifty years. Attitudes about work, play, relationships, and self inform how we come together and stay together. Family is not necessarily defined by biological connections; many of us choose our families, or are chosen.

In the context of caregiving, it is important to understand how the changes in the family unit impact the journey of caring for each other. We know that our family systems are important factors in how we age. People with supportive families are known to live longer and experience a better quality of life than those who feel isolated and alone. But sometimes it is not obvious who will care for whom. Who is responsible for care? Who is available to care? Who wants to care? Who is capable of providing care? And who do you want as your caregiver? These questions are incredibly important to consider *before* the caregiving crisis lands on your doorstep.

"Family" Can Be a Loaded Term

Upon completion of a workshop about caregiving, a woman approached me with a wonderful insight. As a self-described orphan, she felt excluded whenever I used the term "family." She was an only child. Unmarried. And her parents were both deceased. She did not have a family based upon her limited understanding of the term, a biological connection or legally recognized union. As I explained my broader definition of family, her eyes filled with tears. She no longer felt excluded from the conversation. She was not an anomaly in the world. For all future programs, she suggested that I explain my usage of the term "family" to ensure that everyone felt included in the conversation. Rest assured, I do.

Pure Genius!

Regardless of how you choose to define your family, there is a foundational truth about all families that we must embrace. *All* families are dysfunctional at some level. Families are not about perfection. Never have been. Never will be. Yet we often expect perfection, particularly during the most stressful times. We are supposed to rise to the occasion, right? Well, the reality is that any family system under enough stress will manifest dysfunctional behaviors. So I encourage all of us to have realistic expectations and be gentle with ourselves and our families during the times that try our souls. The journey of caregiving is hard enough. We need not make it harder by expecting the impossible from our families.

The Evolution of the Family System

Before we jump into the topic of family systems evolution, I want to ensure that everyone feels included in the conversation. The term "family" implies different things to different people. When I refer to your family, I attach no qualifiers or stipulations to the term. Family does not necessarily mean a biological connection. Nor does the term indicate a legally recognized union of two people. For our purposes, *family* is defined by *you*. This could be your family of origin or perhaps your family of choice. Maybe a lovely mix of the two. Regardless, consider yourself included in the conversation about families.

You need not be an expert in the social sciences to realize that the family unit has changed dramatically over the past fifty to seventy-five years in the United States. The transformation of the family should come as no surprise. Life is evolutionary. Now, wait. I am not opening a Darwinian can of worms. I merely want to establish the fact that life is a continuous process of change. Our social structures reflect societal and cultural norms, which are predicated on individual beliefs, values, and principles. Our social structures (families) change as we change. Thus, our family units represent generational attitudes, perspectives, and characteristics. The traditional family of my parents' generation reflected their generational values. Today, the various forms of family units reflect the values of Boomers and the younger generations.

Traditional Family

A family unit composed of a husband, a wife, and children. The husband is the financial support for the family. Obviously, this term is somewhat dated!

Definition

If you recall, we listed the notable characteristics of the Boomer generation in **Chapter 1**. Take a moment and review the list. Now, let's consider the characteristics of family units today and see if there is a correlation. Families today are:

- smaller than previous generations;
- often single-person units;
- geographically dispersed;
- two-income families;
- blended (remarriage);
- mobile;

- cohabiting couples;

- same-sex couples;

- nonsexual couples;

- biracial;

- multicultural;

- multifaith;

- multigenerational.

Many of the characteristics associated with family units today reflect societal changes, financial concerns, and technological advances. However, many of the family units reflect generational attitudes and values (i.e., two-income families, same-sex couples, etc.). What is important for our discussion is to recognize how the transformation of the traditional family helps and/or hinders our ability to care for each other.

In **Part 2**, we will review a rigorous assessment process that identifies caregiving needs, wants, goals, and resources. So I will save that discussion for later. But, in regard to family units, I would like to highlight the typical concerns and issues associated with the family structure. Consider the following scenarios:

- There is a growing trend in the United States to "go solo"—to live alone. This has obvious implications for caregiving. If you are ill or incapacitated, who will care for you?

- For families choosing not to have children or for geographically dispersed families, there is a similar concern of who will care for the aging members. Geographic proximity is a complicating factor for most families because our society is transient. Long-distance caregiving typically complicates and magnifies the stress for families.

- Alternative lifestyles—cohabiting, nonsexual, or same-sex couples— can lead to legal complications. In those situations, documentation of wishes and legal designation of a health care agent are critically important.

Divorce is not an uncommon or stigmatized situation for Boomers. Subsequently, many Boomers remarry and establish new family units. Blended families are quite common—two adults from previous marriages (with children) coming together to create a new family. New designations emerge. Stepchild. Stepparent. Ex-spouse. Ex-partner. All is well until a health care crisis occurs. Too often the family discovers that advance directives have not been updated or, even more tragically, were never completed. This can lead to nasty disagreements and legal battles related to end-of-life care. You are well advised to review all your documents when transitioning from one relationship to another to ensure beneficiaries, powers of attorney, and advance directives are current.

Uninspired

Plan for the Unexpected

Several years ago, I learned of a tragic situation that highlights the importance of planning and documentation. A colleague related the story of a lesbian couple confronted by a medical emergency, legal restrictions, and resistant family members. Pat and Joan had been partners for fifteen years and enjoyed an incredible relationship despite the objections of both their families. Pat had suffered a massive stroke and was on life support for ten days while the family struggled to make the needed decisions. Because Pat did not have an advance directive, a medical power of attorney, and HIPAA release forms, her partner of fifteen years was excluded from the end-of-life discussions. Furthermore, Pat's family prohibited Joan from seeing Pat in the intensive care unit. Joan was not present at the bedside when Pat died or at the funeral. As I listened to the story, my heart broke for these women. This was a once-in-a-lifetime moment—the end of life. It didn't have to be a time of confrontation, legal maneuvering, and heated debate. With the required documentation, Joan could have enjoyed the legal status necessary to implement Pat's wishes and to remain by her side until death. Lesson learned. Life doesn't always go as planned. Pat never imagined suffering a massive stroke. She didn't realize the risks of procrastination. Sadly, she and Joan suffered the consequences of her inaction.

Leave Your Ego and Title at the Door

Clara was absolutely distraught. A week ago, she received a call from the police relating the tragic news that her husband, Sam, had been critically injured in a car wreck. Since then, she learned more about traumatic brain injuries than she ever wanted to know. She also learned that Sam had failed to update his advance directives since his previous marriage. Sam's ex-wife, Amanda, was the designated health care agent with the legal right to make decisions for Sam.

Clara met Amanda years ago at a family function, the graduation of one of the children. She seemed nice enough at the time. However, things were quite different today. Could this be any harder? She was furious with Sam. How could he be so thoughtless? How could he do this to her? Clara raged against the fates and allowed herself the luxury of a good cry. Once done, she knew what she must do—call Amanda.

Amanda was surprised to hear from Clara and immediately knew something must be wrong. Upon hearing the news, she expressed her sympathies to Clara. Amanda was even more surprised to learn that she was listed as the health care agent for Sam. However, Sam was never good with details. Kind of an awkward situation, eh? The wife and ex-wife discussing health care options for their guy? Most men would not be quite so trusting! But back to reality. Amanda and Clara decided to meet and discuss their options. You might be amazed by how these women ultimately decided to address the situation. They left their egos and titles at the door.

Fast forward one year. Clara and Amanda decided to join forces. It mattered not who was the ex-wife, the current wife, or the legally recognized health care agent. Sam needed them both. The past was the past. They needed to focus on the task at hand. Amanda and Clara worked collaboratively throughout the crisis and recovery period. Together, they met with doctors, therapists, and counselors. They regularly updated Sam's children (from both marriages), discussed the prognosis, and created an atmosphere of cooperation and caring. As a result, a situation that had the potential to divide and conquer a family served to strengthen the ties that bind. Bravo, ladies!

The Importance of Family

The importance of our social support systems cannot be stressed enough. We know that our families, friends, coworkers, and peers are a factor in successful aging. These are the people who share the good times, and the bad, with us. The ups and the downs. The celebrations and the fights. Our families serve as the inner circle, our intimate relationships that support and sustain us. Our families are typically the first line of defense when we are challenged by aging, illness, and associated disabilities. This is our comfort zone. Trusted. Known.

Family also provides a sense of belonging, that incredible feeling of "being at home." Home has always been important to me. My mom was *the* best at creating a space where all felt welcomed and embraced—family, friends, and strangers. Growing up, our home was the gathering place. From this incredible foundation, I engaged and explored life. It mattered not where I wandered. Ultimately, I longed to go home and reconnect with my roots—to experience that incredible sense of belonging.

I was twenty-four years old when my mom died. Upon her death, I not only lost my mom, I lost my sense of home. I was devastated. Lost. Adrift. At the time, I was also terrified. I had never been without that grounding, reassuring sense of belonging. I ached to go home once again. Now, thirty-two years later, I recognize that same ache in people who have been displaced from their homes as a consequence of aging, illness, and/or disability. As I listen to the stories of people who moved from their homes into long-term care communities, I hear the sadness in their voices and see the fear in their eyes. Many long-term care communities are lovely, offering a variety of programs, services, and amenities. But, it's *not* home! Home is where the heart is. We long to be surrounded by our stuff, our people, and—in my case— our critters.

In our increasingly transient society, it is important to recognize our fundamental need and desire for "home." Too often, we fail to recognize the loss and grief caused by the transitions prompted by aging and illness. When everything else is beyond our control (physical or cognitive decline), our sense of home provides the needed foundation from which to confront

Going Home

One of the greatest blessings of my seminary experience was meeting Kay. Our paths crossed in 2003, and we have become forever friends and family over the past decade. Kay is eleven years my senior, a fact I like to highlight from time to time! However, her seniority serves me well. Kay provides a sneak preview of the challenges, opportunities, questions, and choices I will encounter over the next ten to twenty years. Her decision-making process reveals her priorities in life—family and home.

Several years ago, Kay recognized that she had a decision to make. Living in the foothills west of Denver, she realized she wasn't getting any younger. Winters were becoming increasingly problematic. The drive into Denver was not getting any shorter. And the remoteness of her home was becoming a burden instead of blessing. So she explored various parts of the country to determine *the* best place to land. For several years, we discussed the pros and cons of various places. Since I had a vested interest in her decision—a new vacation spot—I enthusiastically supported locations with sunshine, warm temps, beaches, and golf courses. So imagine my disappointment when Kay shared that she had decided to move to Wisconsin! Wisconsin? Not *even* on my radar screen!

Now if you are from Wisconsin, please know I am not disparaging your state. I am originally from Texas. My blood is just too thin for Wisconsin winters. But this is not about me. Back to Kay. Why Wisconsin? Well, Wisconsin is home to Kay. She was born and raised there. She still has family in Wisconsin. And generations of her family lived and died in Wisconsin. She felt compelled to return to her roots. She longed to belong. She wanted to go home. And so she did. Initially, Wisconsin made no sense to me. But now, having witnessed and supported Kay's transition back home, it makes all the sense in the world. Dorothy had it right. There is no place like home.

the challenges of life. So, whether caregiver or care receiver, be mindful of the importance of home and family. This awareness will enhance your compassion and extend your capacity to care for others.

Who Will Care for Me?

As we age, we become more reflective about life and also about death. Perhaps it is because the horizon seems a bit closer than when we were in our twenties and thirties. Personally, I think it a good thing to be mindful of the finitude of life. An awareness that life is limited enhances our appreciation of the moment. We can also be motivated to proactively plan for the eventuality that we will become care receivers. Although this may sound like a morbid and depressing endeavor, it doesn't have to be.

Don't Expect Perfection

Caregiving in the twenty-first century is essentially different from caregiving in the early twentieth century for a variety of reasons:

- We live longer.

- We require higher levels of care for longer periods of time.

- Families are smaller. Fewer hands to provide the needed care.

- Families are geographically dispersed and highly mobile.

- The majority of women are employed outside the home.

- Medical advances afford medications and interventions never before imagined.

- The majority of people die of complications associated with chronic conditions rather than acute illnesses.

- The increased incidence of Alzheimer's disease strains family systems and long-term care service providers.

- Family units vary greatly, with some types being more accommodating to the long-term care needs of the aging and/or ill.

- Our health care system transferred much of the responsibility of recovery and care to families, often with little training or preparation.

Planning to Get Old(er) and Weird(er)

Several years ago, my best friend and I had a moment of inspiration that led to a life-changing decision. JoAnne and I decided to get old(er) and weird(er)—together! At the time, we had been friends for many years and spent the majority of our leisure time together. JoAnne is the sister I never had. So, as we discussed previously, JoAnne is my "chosen" family. We also thought it a good idea to invite other friends who were also single and concerned about the aging process. Bottom line, if you are single (for whatever reason), have no children, or choose not to rely on your children as you age, you'd better have a plan. You need a plan that affords the opportunity to create a life-giving community in which to grow old. Do not assume a plan will come together and all will be well. Perhaps it is the control queen in me, but I want to have a voice in how I will age—with whom, where, how, and when!

I am blessed to have amazing friends whom I have met over the course of my lifetime. Women from all walks of life. These ladies are my dearest friends, my family of choice. Over the years, our paths crossed in a variety of places for a variety of reasons. Childhood friends. Colleagues. A fellow seminarian. Church family. Regardless of how or where we met, these women are my family, always and forever. This is the group in which I feel "at home." I have no doubt that I belong. Thank goodness my friends feel the same way. After much discussion, research, laughter, and debate, we decided to get old(er) and weird(er) together! We committed to completing this journey together. And we intend to have as much fun as possible along the way.

So we are gradually implementing our plan of consolidation. We will ultimately live together—sharing expenses, sharing the journey, and sharing ourselves. We will support each other physically, emotionally, and spiritually. When the time comes, we will share in the expense of home health care. However, there is one piece of the puzzle we are actively seeking. We want to recruit younger versions of ourselves, probably twenty years our junior. These people will have the delight of living with an amazing group of women for *free*. In return, we ask that these younger people open our pill bottles, get us out and about, and pour a lovely glass of wine from time to time! I can guarantee there will never be a dull moment in our home!

I relate this story somewhat tongue in cheek. But in reality, this is our plan and our dream. Aging with the people you know the best and love the most! I am no longer worried about who will care for me. My family will be there for me. And I will be there for them. If you are wondering who will care for you, feel free to take our idea and run with it. May your intentional community of care serve you well.

Today's journey of caregiving looks and *feels* quite different from that of previous generations. Everything seems to be magnified in the twenty-first century. *Higher* levels of care. *Longer* durations of care. *More* complex disease processes. *Increased* expenses. *Fewer* resources. *Enhanced* sense of isolation. Responding to the changes posed by aging and illness is one of the most stressful times within a family. So have realistic expectations of yourself and your family. Caregiving is not about perfection. More often than not, caregiving is about showing up, being present, and taking one step at a time. In this regard, the essence of caregiving is timeless.

To Summarize...

🔍 There is no "traditional" family in the United States today. Our families come in all shapes and sizes. The evolution of the family system over the past fifty to seventy-five years has direct implications on how we care for each other. It is important to recognize the potential challenges posed by the journey of caregiving and assess your family's ability to respond to the call for care.

🔍 Remind Toto, "There is no place like home."

🔍 To achieve our desired sense of belonging as we age, we must be proactive, and perhaps creative, in developing a support community. Ask yourself the question "Who will care for me?" If there is no obvious answer, you know what to do! Call, email, text, Tweet, or track down the people you love the most. Invite them to get old(er) and weird(er) *with* you. How could they resist such a tantalizing invitation?

🔍 Caregiving can be a trial for all involved. So don't expect the process to be perfect. Don't expect your family to respond perfectly. Be gentle with yourself and your family. One step at a time, the journey of caregiving transforms one and all.

Chapter 3

Change Is the Norm: Deal with It!

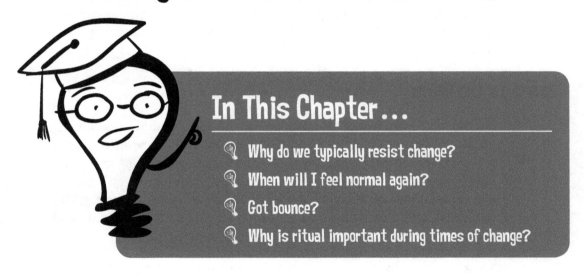

In This Chapter...

- 💡 Why do we typically resist change?
- 💡 When will I feel normal again?
- 💡 Got bounce?
- 💡 Why is ritual important during times of change?

Our expectations of life inform our responses to change. Life is a continuous process of change. Yet we act as if change is an aberration! We become defensive, angry, resistant, and downright ornery when change occurs. Why? We are creatures of habit. We love the known. We relish our routines. Consequently, anything that deviates from the norm threatens our sense of normalcy. So when life changes suddenly, or even gradually, we resist. We defend the status quo with every fiber of our being.

Aging results in a variety of changes—anticipated and unexpected. The normal process of aging results in physical and cognitive changes. With the advent of illness, the process of aging accelerates and the repercussions ripple throughout the family system. To understand our reactions to change, we must understand the process of change and transition. Granted, unwanted and unexpected change will persist in rocking the boat on occasion. But I believe that knowledge of the process prepares us well for the ripples and waves in life.

Aging, illness, and disability prompt countless changes in our lives—most uninvited and unwelcome. Although we cannot control everything that happens in our lives, we always retain the freedom to choose an attitude in response to the change(s). Our choice directly impacts our lived experience and quality of life. Recognition of this choice in the midst of change transforms the victimizing question of "Why?" into the empowering inquiry of "What now?" This is particularly important when confronted by the ultimate change—death.

Change Is the Norm

Do you welcome change? This is a question I pose to audiences when I present programs on change and transition. Usually, there are a few brave souls who boldly proclaim they welcome change. Change is invigorating! Then there are a few people who want to qualify their answers. They like certain kinds of change, but not all change. A discerning group! The remaining majority of the audience nervously wiggles around in their chairs, staring at the ground. Change is daunting for most of us.

Most human beings are not fond of change, invited or not. Change disrupts our daily routines, life expectations, and sense of certainty. Change reminds us that we are not in control! But change is a given in life: the seasons change, society changes, financial markets change, relationships change, and we change. So instead of resisting change, how can we engage it? How can we integrate change into our lives?

We would be better served if we entered the world with realistic expectations. In delivery rooms throughout the country, a standard piece of equipment should be a sign that states, "Change Ahead." In fact, the message could be embroidered on the masks of the OB/GYN staff—a more intimate, personalized message. I would have certainly appreciated the heads up (no pun intended) after popping out of the womb and taking my first breath. But, then, I have always been a planner! When planning a road trip, I check road conditions for the proposed route. If there is construction, a bridge down, or paving projects, I make the needed course adjustments to ensure an enjoyable trip. The same is true for the journey of life. If I anticipate bumps in the road, I can make a course correction. So it makes sense to have an initial sign indicating what we can expect on this journey of life. Change ahead! Now, you may think this idea silly, but our expectations of life inform our responses to change. We need to have realistic expectations of life. Change *will* happen. So hang on, my friends! Based on my experience, life is a monster roller-coaster ride.

Change is neither good nor bad. Change is merely a deviation from the norm. It is the meaning we ascribe to change that deems it positive or negative. However, we need to realize that even "positive" change is disruptive. Let's say you accept a fabulous promotion offered by your company. More money. More responsibility. More opportunity. All good things, right? Well, all good things except the stipulation that you (and your family) have to move from the West Coast to the East Coast. Ouch! So even positive change serves to disrupt life in challenging ways.

The arrival of change varies as well. Some change is shocking! You receive a call at 3:00 a.m. apprising you that your mother had a stroke. *Wham*! Change just landed in the middle of your living room. Or, perhaps, you await change; you know change is imminent. Such is the case with a progressive illness such as Alzheimer's disease. Every day, you notice one more thing that your mother can no longer remember, one more aspect of life that eludes her. Whether sudden or anticipated, change is daunting. It is daunting because we love our sense of normal. We take comfort in believing we are in control (although the reality is that we rarely are). So when change happens, we desperately hang on to the status quo, the known. We dig in our heels, fortify the walls, and resist the change with all our might.

Our resistance to change is rooted in our fear of the unknown. Human beings don't do well "not knowing." We take great comfort in knowing what is around the corner, knowing what to expect. We love certainty! But the journey of life is by nature mysterious! Remember, aging is a continuous process of change. So we have a choice in how we engage the journey. Will we be paralyzed by our fear of the unknown? Will we resist anything that

In an Instant

There are moments in life when our lives change in a heartbeat—for better or for worse. Even decades later, we can recall those moments with uncanny clarity. It was a sunny, spring day in West Texas. I was fifteen years old. My dad and I were standing in the living room. I remember the sunlight coming through the windows. My cat rubbed against my legs as a constant reminder that I was not alone. I realized that my dad suddenly looked old and weary. He didn't seem sure of himself. He refused to look at me. Instead, his gaze focused on some distant point outside. I can't remember anything he said except for the word "cancer." My mom had breast cancer. Even at that relatively young age, I realized my life had changed forever. At the time, I didn't fully appreciate the implications of cancer for my family (thank goodness). But I did recognize in that moment what I had lost—my childhood. On an unremarkable, spring day in West Texas, one word changed my life forever.

Example

deviates from the norm and thereby become stagnant? Or will we choose to be fascinated by change? Are we willing to relinquish our limiting need for certainty in order to risk exploring the possibilities afforded by change? Transformation and growth entail risk, a required risk if we are to successfully navigate change and live into our full potential. William Bridges, a well-known American author and organizational consultant, stressed the importance of understanding transitions within the context of organizational evolution (*Transitions: Making Sense of Life's Changes, 2004*). A very different setting from that of caregiving; however, the process of change and transition is similar.

Change, within the context of caregiving, comes in a variety of guises. Aging and illness precipitate physical and cognitive changes. These changes then generate other changes: role changes, financial changes, spiritual changes, changes in residence, and changes in hopes and dreams. We noted previously that all change (positive or negative) serves to disrupt life. However, the changes that arrive uninvited, unwanted, and unexpected are particularly challenging. You could argue that we *should* anticipate the changes associated with normal aging. It is a given, a known. As we age, we will change physically and cognitively. However, remember, we live in an age-denying society. We don't want to accept the fact that we are getting older! So how we *should* respond and how we *do* respond are often quite different.

We need to recognize the elephant in the room when it comes to change and caregiving. The ultimate, daunting change is death. And, yes, we will all ultimately die. Yet we live in a death-averse society. We don't want to acknowledge that we are finite creatures with expiration dates. Instead, we choose to focus on how to retain our youth, at all costs! We spend billions

In Order to Succeed, You Must Be Willing to Fail

When I graduated from college (the first time), I began a career in the petroleum business as an exploration geologist. Fresh out of college, the learning curve was steep! I had the added pressure of being one of the few women in the profession at the time. So I felt I had to run faster and jump higher than my male counterparts. I was blessed to have an incredible mentor in the form of my first boss. He not only taught me about the business of petroleum exploration, but he also taught me how to accept the inherent risk of my chosen profession. Don't worry, I won't bore you with the details. Simply put, the odds of drilling a successful exploratory well are between 5 and 10 percent because of all the "unknowns." Just knowing that tidbit of information about the oil business, you can appreciate my angst when considering the likely outcome of my first well. I would fail. My boss picked up on my fear and set me straight. He said exploratory wells were inherently risky. Just the nature of the beast. But if I became paralyzed by my fear of failure, I would never have the opportunity to drill a discovery well. I would never have the chance to succeed. Turns out my boss was a very wise man. I ultimately drilled my fair share of dry holes. However, I also drilled several significant discovery wells because I overcame my fear of failure.

Whether confronted by the challenges of exploration geology or aging, fear of the unknown is our greatest disability. In both situations, we must discover the courage to explore life if we are ever to savor the sweetness of success.

of dollars on cosmetics, age-defying lotions, surgical procedures, and supplements to maintain the illusion of youth. We fight the ravages of gravity by pulling back, lifting up, and tucking in. Gray is not the new black! And if you are feeling a bit deflated by life, there are options to inflate and plump up various parts of the body in amazing ways. Now, with that said, please know that I am as vain as the next person. I pluck gray hairs. Frown at my wrinkles. And lament the southward migration of my body! However, when we obsess on the facade, we fail to appreciate the wholeness of life—mind, body, and spirit. Instead, we live in a state of denial, frantically hiding the evidence of advancing age. By doing so, we miss the opportunity to proactively plan for our ultimate demise. Preparing for the ultimate change (death) frees us to live fully.

Confronting our fear of death would serve our society well in a variety of ways. We will explore this idea to a greater extent in **Chapter 20**.

Longing for Normal

Why is change so destabilizing? Well, in order to understand our reaction (or resistance) to change, we need to understand the process of change. Then it will all become clear! Change, by definition, means that something ends and something new begins. For example, let's say you decide to change jobs. You tender your letter of resignation and accept a new job. There will be a period of adjustment—a transition—from the moment of resignation until you settle in at your new job. Even though you wanted this new job, you feel anxious and uncertain. You are going to miss your former colleagues. You will stay in touch. But it won't be the same as seeing them every day. Naturally, you will miss them. Although the new job seems perfect, you start to question your decision. What if your new boss turns out to be a nightmare? What if you made a mistake? Well, too late now. You resigned. No turning back.

When change happens (by choice or because of circumstances), we feel disconnected from the normal and the known. Consequently, we feel unsettled, anxious, and fearful. We are in unknown territory! Nothing looks familiar. We don't know what to expect. And we desperately seek our comfort zone. We want to go back! We long to feel normal again. However, the reality is that we can't go back. We must determine how best to proceed, establish a new normal, and embrace a new beginning.

An image is truly worth a thousand words (or maybe more). So I would like to offer an image that reflects the process of change. Imagine your life as a journey. The path is smooth and level, until something happens. *Change*! This change is represented by the entrance to a bridge. The bridge serves to transport you over the rough waters stirred up by the change in your life. The bridge is narrow, allowing travel only in one direction. Once on the bridge, you realize you can't go back. You start to panic! The other side of the bridge vanishes in a thick bank of fog. What is on the other side of this bridge? You want to know where you are going, but your efforts prove futile. You can't see

Example

I Want to Feel Normal Again

"I just want to feel normal again." Poignant words I recall my mom saying almost forty years ago. We were sitting on the couch in our den; my mom was leaning against me. Over the past forty-eight hours, we had been through hell and back following a particularly difficult round of chemotherapy. As her caregiver (and daughter), I had been by her side the entire time. We were through the worst of the physical side effects of the treatment, but the emotional pain lingered. Looking out the windows, we realized it was a glorious spring day. I could sense the overwhelming sadness in my mom. She wanted to be in her gardens—planting flowers, pruning bushes, and digging dandelions. My mom rarely complained or whined over the course of eight years of surgeries, chemotherapy, and radiation treatments. But today, it was the simplest of things that caused her to proclaim, "I just want to feel normal again!" As I held my mom and shared in her desire for normalcy, I learned to appreciate the small things in life. It is not the *extra*ordinary things in life that sustain us. Rather, it is our sense of the sacred discovered in the simplest of things that keeps us afloat during the times that try our souls.

It is the simple things in life that give us that reassuring sense of normalcy. Therefore, it is the simple things in life we long for when confronted by significant change and transition. Today, whenever I need a dose of normalcy, I head out to the backyard and dig up some dandelions. Simple, yet sacred.

that far ahead. So there you stand. You can't return to your former life. You have no idea what the future holds. And the bridge is the only option you have if you choose to continue your journey. Although frightening, the bridge offers the hope of a new beginning. Will you find the courage to walk into the unknown? Or will you allow fear to abbreviate your journey? The choice is yours.

Our experience of change and transition depends on the attitude we *choose*. Yes, it is a choice. In the midst of change and transition, so many things are beyond our control. It is nice to realize that we have control over something! I can't control everything that happens in my life (much to my dismay). However, I always have a choice in how I choose to respond. This is not a novel approach to life or a recent revelation. Famous and not-so-famous people share this foundational belief. I am an ardent student and fan of Viktor Frankl, the twentieth-century psychologist and Holocaust survivor who eloquently discusses the importance of attitude in his classic book, *Man's Search for Meaning*. By the way, if you have not read this book, you must! Frankl serves to remind all of us that we not only have the freedom to choose an attitude when challenged by life, but we also have the responsibility. How do we choose to respond to life? An important question to ponder. We need not be victims of change, stranded on the bridge. We can choose to walk across and reengage with life.

Having described the bridge as a metaphor for change, it's obvious that we don't fear change as much as we fear the transitional period *after* change. Sometimes we aren't even aware that change is about to happen. So there is no opportunity to fear the looming change. This is very important to recognize and appreciate if we are to manage change well. Change happens, and we find ourselves on the bridge before we know it. This is the time of uncertainty. The fog rolls in, clouding our perspective of life. Perhaps we've never been on this bridge before. Is it structurally sound? Are the boards strong or rotten? Can the bridge be trusted to carry us over the chasm of raging water? Good questions to ask. But don't hold your breath waiting for reassuring answers! To move on with your life often requires a leap of faith. Choosing to walk across the transitional bridge requires courage, determination, hope, and faith. Not your typical walk in the park!

The transitional bridge also serves as a platform for grief and mourning. Change, by definition, means that something ends and something new

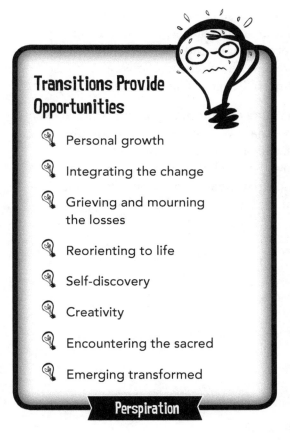

Transitions Provide Opportunities

- Personal growth
- Integrating the change
- Grieving and mourning the losses
- Reorienting to life
- Self-discovery
- Creativity
- Encountering the sacred
- Emerging transformed

Perspiration

begins. With every ending comes a sense of loss and our need to grieve that loss. As in the previous example of changing jobs, there are lost relationships and routines. Within the context of aging and illness, we experience the loss of good health, loss of youth, loss of cognitive and physical abilities, loss of home, loss of loved ones, and on and on. There is a tremendous amount of loss to be addressed, processed, and integrated into the fabric of our beings. Before moving forward, we must grieve and mourn our losses. We cannot embrace a new beginning until we bid adieu to the past. No wonder change and the resultant transitions are daunting!

Bouncing Is a Choice

From the perspective of caregivers and care receivers, the issue of change is a daily challenge and concern. Over the course of a progressive, degenerative illness, families navigate a myriad of changes: physical, cognitive, emotional, psychosocial, spiritual, financial, and logistical. It amazes me just how much change individuals and families endure over the course of a lifetime. We are often more resilient than we ever imagined. We rise to the occasion. We bounce back! How is that possible? Well, the reality is this. We have a choice in the matter. We *choose* to bounce! And the ability to bounce is rooted in our perspective of life and our connection to life-sustaining support (family, friends, and faith).

At birth, I think we should all be issued a set of heavy-duty shock absorbers with detailed instructions on how and when to use. I know of no one who has been able to avoid the bumps and resultant bruises of life. As human beings, we will experience the highs and lows of life—and the transitions between the peaks and valleys are rough. It is during the stressful, difficult times that we realize the importance of resilience—the ability to bounce back from adversity. *Resilience* is not a trait. Rather, it is a process of adaptation. Life can be shocking, to say the very least! Instead of being shattered by the unexpected and the unwanted, we have the ability to choose a response to change. To meet the most daunting challenges of life, we gotta have bounce!

The good news is that resilience is quite common. Consider historical events such as the Holocaust, 9/11, the Vietnam War, and recent natural disasters. Consider your friends, neighbors, colleagues, and community. Look in the mirror! Bounce is common! We are resilient beings. And thank goodness for that, because we need resilience to navigate change and transition. The common elements needed to bounce back include the following:

- Optimism
- Courage
- Self-knowledge
- Spiritual practice
- Supportive community
- Resilience role models
- Physical well-being
- Mental and emotional well-being
- Cognitive and emotional flexibility
- Sense of purpose
- Acceptance of change
- Recognition of what is within our control
- Choosing to focus on "What next?" instead of "Why me?"

Ritual in the Midst of Change

Our reactions to change cover the gamut of emotions—fear, excitement, hope, devastation, delight, etc. Whether welcome or not, change prompts an ending with the possibility of a new beginning. Between the ending and the new

Perspiration

Resilience Is Grand Indeed!

When I was sixteen years old, my parents and I hiked the Grand Canyon. Even forty years ago, you were required to have a permit to camp on the floor of the canyon. A fact my dad was unaware of prior to planning our trip. We arrived at the south rim of the canyon eager to hike down, camp for two days, and hike back out. Imagine our chagrin when the park ranger informed us we could not camp on the floor of the canyon! There were no permits available. We then had two options. First, we could enjoy the canyon vicariously from the rim. Second, we could hike down and back in one day. Not to be detoured by a slight variance in our plans, we opted to hike the canyon in one day!

It was an amazing day indeed. We left the rim of the canyon at 4:00 a.m. with a bit of snow falling. By the time we reached the plateau overlooking the Colorado River five hours later, we were enjoying lovely summer-like temperatures and brilliant sunshine. My dad, who was a geologist by trade, regaled us with the geologic history of the Grand Canyon as we walked down the trail. My mom shared her knowledge of desert vegetation and wildlife. And I spent the entire time marveling at the courage and strength of my mom.

A year before, my mom had a unilateral mastectomy following a positive breast biopsy. Subsequent to her surgery, she underwent a series of radiation treatments, which reduced her physical stamina for many months. Needless to say, I was concerned about her ability to complete the hike. However, with each step taken that glorious day, my concerns faded as my mom bounced down the Bright Angel Trail. On that day in the Grand Canyon, my mom chose to embrace the moment. She didn't use her medical condition as an excuse to opt out of the arduous hike. She never complained en route. Instead, she greeted the day with a brilliant smile and grateful heart. She engaged the journey, one step at a time. Down and back. When we finally emerged from the canyon, fifteen hours after we began, my mom was leading the charge! She literally *bounced* out of the canyon! In that moment, I knew what it meant to be courageous, determined, and resilient. That day in the Grand Canyon, I realized that I need *never* be a victim of circumstances. I can choose to bounce back from adversity and reclaim my foundational belief that life is *grand*! In the subsequent forty years, that lesson has served me well. Thanks, Mom!

beginning is the time of transition, a challenging if not frightening time for most. It is during the transitional period that we often feel disconnected and lost. A scary time indeed. So I would like to offer a suggestion, a way in which to reconnect and regain our bearings as we navigate the transitions of life. Ritual.

So what serves to anchor us during times of transition? Well, what do we long for when navigating transitions prompted by change? Think back to the bridge. Don't we long for the familiar? Absolutely! We long to feel normal again. We desperately want to feel comfortable, certain about what is around the next bend of our journey. There is no better way to regain a sense of normalcy and familiarity than through ritual, a process known to you and often practiced countless times. Please know, when I say ritual, I am referring to spiritual and secular, communal and individual, as well as traditional and contemporary practices. Ritual comes in all shapes and sizes. Formal and informal. Ritual can take two hours or two seconds. I understand ritual in the broadest sense of the term. There is no need to limit ritual to a religious or spiritual context for the purpose of this discussion. If the process serves as a conduit for connection, provides meaning, and touches your heart—it is ritual indeed!

Ritual is described as a prescribed set of actions involving symbolic elements. The purpose of ritual is to provide a sense of continuity, connection, and meaning for those engaged in the process. Ritual provides a sense of certainty, normalcy, and predictability that we need and want when everything else is beyond our control. During times of change and transition, we hunger for ritual because it assures us that some things do *not* change! Beyond the definition, we know ritual when we see it. We know it when we feel it. Ritual speaks to our hearts and souls; ritual enriches our lives. Consequently, ritual requires that we engage in the process—mind, body, and spirit. Ritual is *much* more than a mere routine. Ritual frames ordinary time as *extra*ordinary time. There is an intention when engaged in ritual that is lacking in a daily routine.

Rituals serve as the needed conduits to connect us to that which sustains and nurtures us during times of change and transition. Rituals serve to connect us to:

 our sense of the divine;

 memories;

- community;

- a particular person;

- hope;

- a sense of normalcy.

Ritual versus Routine

What is the difference between a ritual and routine? I can easily distinguish between the two concepts with a simple example, making a cup of tea. Every morning of the world, I awaken and head downstairs to make a cup of tea. As I wait impatiently for the water to boil, I busy myself with the task of feeding our herd of critters. Our dog and cats can be a bit impatient in the mornings as well. We all have our priorities, right? The critters want food. I need caffeine! This is our morning routine. Basic needs are met and life goes on. My intent is to get the day rolling and my eyes open! Nothing more. Nothing less.

Contrast my morning routine with the ritual of brewing a pot of tea. When I feel the need to slow down and reconnect with life, I brew a pot of tea with the intention to reconnect. I use a very special china tea pot. I select a particular china teacup. And I only use Constant Comment tea. As a young girl, I learned this ritual from my mom. When I see the china service and smell the tea, I am transported back in time. Every step in the brewing process is meaningful. Ordinary time becomes *extra*ordinary time. The symbols (teapot, teacup, and tea) are known, familiar, and comforting. The ritual serves as the conduit through which I reconnect with my mom, countless memories, my sense of the divine, and my sense of self.

Hence, if I merely need a jolt of caffeine, routine serves me well. If I long for a heartfelt connection that serves to soothe my soul, nothing less than my time-honored family ritual of brewing a pot of tea will do.

The connections achieved through ritual, subsequently, provide a sense of:

- meaning;
- order;
- certainty;
- comfort;
- healing;
- understanding;
- assurance;
- integration;
- peace.

Rituals employ symbols to represent that which we find difficult to articulate. Symbols evoke responses, provide connections, and convey meaning dependent on your understanding of and experience with the symbol. So something that speaks to my heart may be insignificant to you. Additionally, the meaning of a particular item may be transformed if we choose to see the item differently.

I realize that ritual is a term that serves to alienate some people because of the religious overtones. If you have not been a fan of ritual in the past, I hope that my depiction of ritual serves as an invitation to explore the possibilities afforded by ritual. You need not be ordained, a member of a faith community, or even consider yourself religious to access the benefits and blessings of ritual. On the other hand, if ritual is currently part of your religious and/or spiritual tradition, keep going to the well during times of change and transition. Ritual will provide the connections, the continuity, and the solace you seek.

A Different Kind of Communion

Many years ago, a friend of mine shared the tragic news that her sister, Hannah, had been diagnosed with an inoperable, malignant brain tumor. At the time, Hannah was in her early thirties. She was married, with two young children. Although the odds were against her, she opted to endure aggressive chemotherapy and hoped for a miracle. Every three weeks for a year, Hannah took the prescribed medications followed by a week of debilitating fatigue, nausea, diarrhea, and other nasty side effects. During those very difficult weeks, my friend cared for Hannah and the children. It was obviously hard on Hannah. But it was devastating for her family to witness the process as well.

After nine months of treatment, my friend witnessed something that transformed her perception of chemotherapy. On this particular night, my friend had just put the children to bed. Hannah was in another part of the house preparing to take her regimen of drugs. As my friend walked past Hannah's bathroom, she noticed the door was cracked. She glanced in to make sure all was well only to see Hannah on the floor. Thinking she had fainted or fallen, my friend rushed in to help her. Upon entering, Hannah calmly looked up and smiled. She then invited my friend to kneel with her on the floor. It was then that my friend noticed the pills and a bottle of water on the counter. Confused, but thankful Hannah was okay, she kneeled and asked for an explanation.

Hannah shared that after the second round of chemotherapy, she seriously considered giving up. The side effects were destroying her body and her spirit. But she realized her only hope of living resided in the effectiveness of the drugs. So instead of fighting the drugs, she decided to receive the drugs every three weeks as if it were communion. When she received the chemotherapy treatments, she now welcomed "the elements" into her body. The pills no longer symbolized pain and suffering. Instead, the pills became a sign of hope and long life. Hannah chose to understand the process of chemotherapy differently. Instead of being life threatening and something to reject, chemotherapy had the potential to be life giving and should be embraced! Hannah transformed the meaning of her treatments and thus her attitude about the process.

Rituals often transform the lived experience. But, as Hannah demonstrated, sometimes the lived experience transforms ritual. Hannah employed different elements in the sacred ritual of communion; however, the pills and the water symbolized the same thing to Hannah—hope and salvation. We all see life uniquely. Hannah chose to see possibility and hope in what some considered a hopeless situation. Her ritual provided the meaning, connection, and hope Hannah needed to complete the cycle of treatment and ultimately beat the odds.

To Summarize...

- Life is a continuous process of change. However, we act as if change is the exception instead of the norm. By understanding the process of change and transition, we realize that we are not fearful of and resistant to change. Rather, we are fearful of the transitional period that follows change. The transition is a time of unknowing, uncertainty, and instability. And yet the transitional time is also an opportunity to integrate the change into our lives and discover the courage to move on.

- Change, by definition, means that something ends. When something ends, we experience a sense of loss, which causes us to grieve and mourn. Quite often, this is the time we long to feel normal again. The harsh reality is that we can't go back. We must choose to release the past in order to embrace a new beginning.

- The changes posed by aging and illness are considered *the* most daunting for individuals and families. How do people bounce back from incredible hardship and adversity? Resilience. Resilience is not a trait. It is a process that involves behaviors, actions, and thoughts. Furthermore, resilience is a choice. When challenged by the complexities of aging and illness, we can choose to bounce back.

- During times of change and transition, when nothing seems normal, ritual provides a needed sense of continuity, connection, normalcy, and predictability.

Chapter 4

Caregiving Is a Family Challenge

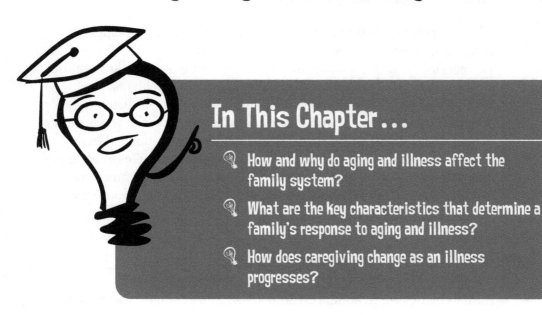

In This Chapter...

- How and why do aging and illness affect the family system?

- What are the key characteristics that determine a family's response to aging and illness?

- How does caregiving change as an illness progresses?

Aging and illness are certainly individual challenges. However, when advanced age and illness bang on the front door, the entire family is awakened by the ruckus! An individual ages. An individual becomes ill. But the family is called to care! We must recognize that illness is *the* most feared and daunting challenge confronted by families. The family system experiences tremendous stress, sometimes for extended periods of time. So have realistic expectations of your family. All families are fundamentally dysfunctional. Don't expect your family to engage the journey of caregiving perfectly!

Within each family, there are rules and expectations that serve as the foundation of a family. From that foundation, we build our unique, quirky clans! The key characteristics of a family (roles, structure and organization, patterns of communication, and foundational beliefs) determine how a family responds and reacts to the challenges of illness and advanced age. By reflecting on the building blocks of your family, you may have an "aha moment." That moment when it all becomes clear! You finally understand *why* your family behaves the way it does when the winds howl and the heavens open up. You recognize predictable patterns of behavior. Some good. Some not so much! Keep in mind, families are not about perfection. Be gentle with yourself and your family.

As noted previously in **Chapter 1**, one of the most daunting aspects of caregiving in the United States today is the duration of caregiving (averaging 4.6 years). Caregiving is not a short-term commitment. Families experience an emotional roller coaster as the challenges of illness ebb and flow. With progressive, ultimately terminal illness, there are predictable stages: diagnosis (acute stage), chronic, remission (in some cases), and terminal. At each stage, illness poses different challenges that mandate different responses from the care receiver and the caregivers. Families must realize that different stages also necessitate different approaches and attitudes. Families learn to relish the occasional plateaus of peace, because they know things can and will change, often without notice.

The Family Challenge of Aging and Illness

Human beings are relational creatures. I visualize human beings as little pieces of Velcro. We attach to each other! It's what we do. It's who we are. We live and thrive in community. I realize some of us are a bit more social than others. But fundamentally, we desire and seek out traveling companions for the journey of life. This mutually beneficial companioning is a boon to one and all. I imagine life as a spectacular spider web that connects everything and everyone! If I sneeze, you'll feel it! If you shiver, I'll be all shook up! Within the web, I have the ability to affect you. And you have the ability to affect me. In very simplistic terms, this is what systems theory is all about. Families are systems. The ripple effects of change (illness and aging) shake everyone up!

Illness and aging are threats to the stability of the family system. Imagine a house of cards. You remove one card, and what happens? The entire structure comes tumbling down, right? The same is true when a family member becomes seriously ill. One person moves out of place, and the family is out of balance. There is a period of readjustment when people scramble to cover the bases and regain their footing. The ability of a family to establish a new balance is dependent on its capacity to adapt, accommodate, and adjust to the changes posed by aging and illness.

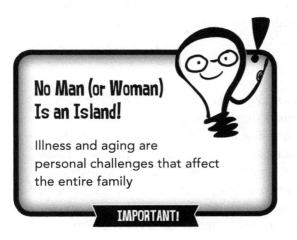

No Man (or Woman) Is an Island!

Illness and aging are personal challenges that affect the entire family

IMPORTANT!

In the midst of rebalancing and rebuilding, we need to realize that family members are emotionally raw. We are not only dealing with logistical issues of family function, but we are also struggling with the reality that someone we love is ill or perhaps dying. The challenge for the family is to meet the immediate demands of the illness while dealing with the unknown aspects of the future.

In the aftermath of a destabilizing event (illness), chaos may reign for a period of time. Not everyone in your family will respond to the crisis in the same way or at the same time. Some will be resistant, longing for normal. Others will be leading the charge to confront the challenge. A few will be shocked and dazed, preferring to live in the land of denial. Quite the challenge to gather this group together and establish a new normal! Very much like herding cats (I know about that which I speak). So, in order to regroup, refocus, and reengage, you must

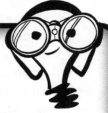

Don't Expect Perfection

Imperfect human beings populate families. A collective of imperfection will not respond perfectly to a crisis! Have realistic expectations of your family.

Observation

understand what makes a family tick, particularly *your* family. What holds your family together? What tears your family apart? Leverage your collective strengths. Recognize and address your collective weaknesses. Understand the process and the resources needed to resurrect your house of cards.

Family Systems in a Nutshell

In the 1970s and 1980s, therapists and counselors had a collective "aha moment." They recognized that individuals must be viewed within the context of the systems in which they live. It seems so obvious, doesn't it? In order to understand an individual and provide wise counsel, you must understand the context in which the person lives. We are not known in isolation; rather, we are known in relationship with others. This is the essence and focus of *family systems theory*. Families are systems of interconnected and interdependent individuals. In order to understand the individual, you must understand the inner workings of the family.

This was a good first step in expanding the perspective of therapeutic interventions. However, there were more improvements yet to come. Many doctors and nurses realized treatment of only the biological concerns was also inadequate; a bridge between the mind and body was essential. To serve patients well, health care providers needed to appreciate the emotional, as well as the biological, impact of illness on the entire family system.

Furthermore, in the 1970s, George Engel recognized the destabilizing effect illness had on families. In fact, Engel described illness as a member of the family. As such, illness impacts not only the person who is ill but also *every* member of the family. Toward the end of the twentieth century, an integrated approach to care emerged that served to humanize health care. Health care providers expanded the scope of service. If the family system in which the patient lived was falling apart due to the ripple effects of illness, then the patient was less likely to thrive. So the family needed to be considered when developing a plan of care, making decisions, and establishing goals. Hallelujah and amen! Caregivers were finally recognized as an integral aspect of care.

So, in a nutshell, this is the *biopsychosocial approach*, which is becoming the standard approach in health care. An essential element (and benefit) of the biopsychosocial approach is the interaction among the patient, family members, and health care providers. It is not a top-down approach to health care with the doctor dictating a plan of care. Instead, it is a collaborative approach that allows for all voices to be heard and all concerns to be addressed. A much more compassionate, effective approach to care, in my humble opinion!

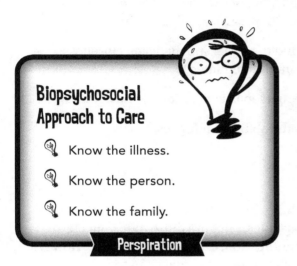

Biopsychosocial Approach to Care

🔧 Know the illness.

🔧 Know the person.

🔧 Know the family.

Perspiration

Key Characteristics of Family Systems

Families are complex systems. Often perplexing, if not downright mysterious. Complex or not, we need to understand how families work (or not) in order to meet the challenges posed by illness and aging. In the middle of a crisis, ignorance is *not* bliss! So let's examine the basic components and attributes common to all families, the basic building blocks of family systems: family structure, roles, communication styles, and family beliefs. Once you know the basics, you can then apply the foundational principles to your specific family system. By doing so, you will discover the hows and whys of your family's response to illness, aging, and caregiving. A good thing indeed!

Family Structure and Organization

If you think about your family as a corporation, you will recognize the importance of an organizational framework. Who reports to whom? Who is in charge? Who makes decisions? This structure is reinforced by family expectations and rules, the family norms. When illness or complications associated with aging enter the family system, the structure of the family is severely tested (depending on the nature of the illness and duration of care required). If the structure of the family system is too rigid, then the family may not be flexible enough to accommodate the changes. If the family structure is too weak, the family may be too unorganized to develop a plan of care. In order to rise to the occasion, the following components and attributes are needed:

- Adaptability—the ability to rebalance responsibilities, roles, and resources following a destabilizing event such as illness.

- Flexibility—the ability and willingness to *bounce back* from adversity (resilience, as discussed in **Chapter 3**). Bend; don't break!

- Cohesion—the ability to find the sweet spot between closeness (enmeshed) and separation (differentiated).

- Healthy boundaries—interpersonal, generational, and community.

- Tolerance for ambiguity—the ability (willingness) to live with uncertainty.

Roles and Responsibilities

Each member of your family assumes or is assigned roles and responsibilities. The more obvious roles/titles are those reflecting our biological relationships: father, mother, son, daughter, sibling, etc. However, we also assume functional roles such as decision maker, patriarch, matriarch, communicator, clown, wild child, perfect child, cook, maid, financial guru, spiritual leader, etc. You may wear many hats in your family. Just depends on your particular situation.

Family roles must be reassigned when illness compromises a person's cognitive and/or physical abilities. Obviously, some role assignments are more problematic than others. So you need to consider the following:

- *Who* is ill? The *who* is critically important and determines the magnitude and extent of disruption.

- *How* long will the person be incapacitated? Are role changes temporary or permanent?

- *Who* can and will assume relinquished roles?

- *How* will roles be reassigned?

- *What* new roles arise as a consequence of illness? Who will assume the new roles?

- *How* will role reversals affect the family?

Illness Generates New Roles—Caregiver and Care Receiver

Jack and Martha are in shock. They are trying to digest the devastating news that Martha has ALS (Lou Gehrig's disease). Just two weeks ago, they were planning a fabulous Alaskan cruise to celebrate their fortieth wedding anniversary. What happened?

Over the course of Martha's illness, Jack and Martha will remain husband and wife. But they also acquired new roles due to the diagnosis. Jack is a caregiver. Martha is a care receiver. Quite often, the new roles of caregiver and care receiver overshadow the intimate roles of husband and wife. Caregiving becomes an all-consuming journey. Consequently, it is important for families to maintain a balance. We need to encourage each other to retain (or sometimes reclaim) the intimate roles we cherish. Other people can help with the daily errands and chores. Only Jack can be Martha's husband. Only Martha can be Jack's wife. Never relinquish your cherished, intimate roles. Those are the relationships that will support and sustain you through the ups and downs of life.

IMPORTANT!

Role changes, sudden or anticipated, shake things up in a family. Some family members may feel burdened by additional responsibilities. Others may feel left out of the process. Depending on the role that needs to be filled, there may be a power struggle of sorts between family members. Progressive illness and extended periods of caregiving require a rebalancing of roles from time to time. So don't get too comfortable. The odds are things will change. Suffice it to say, families need to become adept at juggling and rebalancing.

Boundaries

Every year, I offer a number of programs on personal and professional boundaries. Usually, an organization calls when something has gone wrong. An employee crossed the line and there is a crisis. *Yikes!* Consequently, most people perceive the discussion of boundaries as punitive. If you are currently furrowing your brow or wrinkling your nose, I invite you to see boundaries in a different light. Boundaries are your friend! Boundaries serve you well. Boundaries are fundamental, structural elements needed to support and sustain your family, particularly during times of crisis. So keep reading. I promise this will be painless.

Boundaries provide the framework within which family members function. The importance of boundaries cannot be overstated. Highly functioning, effective family systems establish and maintain boundaries for the following reasons:

- Boundaries distinguish one person from another.

- Boundaries are mutually beneficial.

- Boundaries delineate a buffer zone between people.

- Boundaries establish physical and emotional limits.

- Boundaries assist in establishing realistic expectations.

Boundaries determine how family members relate to one another. They are a determining factor in the overall health and functional ability (or disability) of the family. Families that exhibit significant dysfunction usually have boundary issues. The boundaries are either nonexistent or incredibly rigid. Either way, not good.

Families move along a continuum between closeness (enmeshed) and separateness (differentiated). As with most things in life, either extreme is not healthy. However, when a family system is stressed, the system gravitates to one extreme or the other. Consider an image to reinforce this idea. Imagine a full tube of toothpaste. Take the lid off the tube. Cut a hole in the other end. Place the tube on the floor. Now step in the middle of the tube. What happened? Same thing happens with families under stress. The family squirts out one end of the tube or the other! When pressed, close is not close enough (enmeshed)! Or far is not far enough (differentiated). Most families have a preferred extreme. It's important to recognize a family's preference. Obviously, either extreme is problematic in the midst of the crisis! Enmeshed families have difficulty establishing and maintaining boundaries. Group think reigns. Detached families have difficulty coming together for a common cause. Support is lacking. The goal is to find the sweet spot along the continuum between closeness and separateness that allows the system to respond effectively to the crisis.

The changes and challenges associated with illness, aging, and caregiving affect *all* boundaries within the family. Some boundaries are destroyed.

Others are reinforced. So forewarned is forearmed. When your family is challenged by aging, illness, and/or caregiving, guard your boundaries; an attack is imminent.

Patterns of Communication

Communication is a critical element within family systems during the best of times. However, effective communication is mandatory if families are to meet the daunting challenges of illness, advanced age, and caregiving. Even knowing this, effective communication is often derailed by the best intentions within families. Often this is a consequence of roles, life cycles, and generational patterns of behavior.

For example, a pattern of secrecy concerning my mom's cancer developed out of her desire to protect our family from the pain of her illness. Several years after Mom's mastectomy, I learned by happenstance, from my family doctor, that cancer had been detected in her lymph nodes. So recurrence was inevitable, in his opinion. Even today, I can remember my sense of bewilderment and betrayal. Since this was obviously something I was not supposed to know, I couldn't confront my mom without causing her unnecessary pain. So I remained silent and perpetuated our family legacy of secrecy. While reflection allows for an understanding of my mom's motivation, the emotional scars are incentive enough to end the pattern of silence and secrecy so prevalent in my family.

We noted earlier in this chapter that family members assume various roles. One of the most important roles is that of communicator. This is the person who serves as traffic control for the entire family. Messages and communiqués of all types pop up on the communicator's screen for distribution to other family members. What happens if the communicator in your family becomes ill or incapacitated? How will information be disseminated in an efficient and effective way? How long will the lines of communication be down? Who will assume the role of communicator?

The loss of the family communicator can paralyze a family in the midst of a crisis. The family must establish new lines of communication. Bottlenecks in the flow of information must be identified and resolved. Obviously, a crisis is not prime time to construct a new communication system. However, it happens quite often. It is the wise family indeed that works to establish and maintain several lines of communication. Having a Plan B for critical family infrastructures minimizes the chaotic impact of illness and aging on the family system.

Foundational Beliefs

What does illness *mean* to you and your family? What is the narrative, the story, associated with illness in your family? Do you anticipate a long and healthy life? Is there a family history of cancer, heart disease, or Alzheimer's disease? Is disease perceived as a biological anomaly or as a punishment? Is the situation literally beyond belief and your worldview shattered? Your faith destroyed? Do you rage against the injustice of life? Or do you accept your fate?

As noted previously, illness is *the* most feared and destabilizing event for most families. We feel threatened. The situation is out of control. Nothing seems familiar or normal. And we desperately want to understand. We want to know "Why?" How your family understands illness determines your reaction and response to the challenge. If your family is like most, not everyone is of the same opinion. People understand illness differently based on their expectations of life, spiritual/religious beliefs, life experience, and cultural norms. The meaning given to an illness ultimately informs and influences the attitudes, actions, and reactions of individuals and families in significant, sometimes life-altering, ways.

Different Stages—Different Responses

In **Chapter 3**, I stressed the fact that life is ever changing. Change is the norm. This fundamental truth (one of the few in life) bears repeating when discussing the impact of illness on the family system. When dealing with progressive and/or chronic illnesses, change is the name of the game. Just when a family starts to feel that things are under control, something happens! As the illness progresses or new symptoms arise, the family reacts to meet the new challenge. Depending on the duration of the illness, families become exhausted by this seemingly endless cycle of change and transition.

Families also need to realize that as an illness progresses, different times require different approaches, skills, and responses from the family. What worked well for the family immediately after diagnosis is not possible or

I Deserve It!

I will never forget a heartbreaking story shared by a physician many years ago. She had a patient, thirty-two years of age. During the annual exam, the doctor discovered the woman had early-stage cervical cancer. However, the prognosis was quite good due to early detection. After explaining the diagnosis and proposed plan of care, the doctor was shocked to learn that the patient had no intention of doing anything! She politely thanked the doctor and prepared to leave. The doctor then stressed the importance of treatment. The cancer was potentially fatal if untreated. The patient realized the implications of her decision, but she was adamant. Her decision was final.

The doctor refused to accept the patient's decision. The odds were good that, if treated, this woman could live a long and happy life! So the doctor pressed for an explanation. Finally,

the patient reluctantly revealed that she previously had an affair during a rough time in her marriage. Her husband never suspected her transgression, nor had she confessed. Since then, she had been consumed by guilt. She had no doubt that her cervical cancer was God's will. Cancer was her punishment, and she deserved it! Cancer was her fate, and she accepted it. There was nothing more to be done. With that, she turned and walked out the door.

Now, years later, the memory was still painful for the doctor. However, she was also thankful for having met that remarkable, courageous woman. Although the doctor didn't condone the decision, she honored and respected her patient. Because of her, the doctor practiced medicine differently. She realized it wasn't enough to know how to effectively treat an illness. She must know how to serve the person by understanding what the illness means to the patient and the family. Seek first to understand, then to be understood. Steven Covey would be so proud!

advisable during the chronic stage of the illness. So, as in all things associated with aging and illness, knowledge of the process allows a family to anticipate future needs and plan accordingly.

Progressive illnesses exhibit three developmental stages: acute, chronic, and terminal. During each stage, families react and respond to the illness in different ways. Each stage requires different coping skills.

Without doubt, the diagnosis of a progressive/terminal illness is a challenge and crisis like no other for a family. Yet it is interesting to note that the Chinese symbol for crisis consists of two characters: danger and opportunity. Could it be that there is an opportunity for growth and transformation in the midst of the chaos? *Yes!* However, the possibility of growth and transformation is more likely when families know what to expect. So let's briefly review the challenges and opportunities presented at each stage of the disease process.

Diagnosis, or Acute Stage

During the acute stage of an illness, it is quite common for the family to come together to meet the demands of the crisis. Perhaps you have experienced this in your own family. A crisis occurs, and your family circles the wagons to meet the challenge! At diagnosis, there may be a short period of shock and denial. But when the reality of the situation settles in, families rally to confront the threat.

Frequently during the acute stage, families become overprotective and violate the autonomy of the patient. We care too much! The patient, if competent and willing, should be involved in designing the plan of care, discussing treatment options, etc. Although enmeshment might prove to be an effective coping mechanism during the acute stage, it is potentially damaging to the patient and the family during the chronic stage.

Chronic Stage

The second stage of an illness is the chronic stage. During the acute stage, the family pulls together to meet the challenge of the crisis. As the illness moves into the chronic stage, the patient and the family begin to comprehend the need for role changes, requirements of care, physical and emotional losses,

Hello?

If you ever want to be ignored, put on a hospital gown and hop in a bed. Invite your family to gather round your bedside. Then wait for the doctor to arrive with some important test results. After the initial greetings, the conversation rises to a high level—above your head! The doctor will address the standing family members, overlooking your supine figure. Information will be shared. Questions posed. Decisions made. And plans confirmed. You witness this from the comfort of your bed, turning your head back and forth as if watching an exciting match at Wimbledon. Occasionally, someone may actually ask for your perfunctory approval. But, rest assured, you don't need to worry about a thing. Your family has everything under control.

Hello? Please do not omit the most important person from the conversation—the patient! I realize we want to protect those we love. However, we can become overfunctioning and paternalistic in the process. So please remember to include all interested parties in the important conversations. That includes the person donning the stylish backless gown.

Perspiration

and the fact that "normal" is no longer possible. The family cannot turn back the clock and resume its "normal" routine. Instead, illness is a new member of the family, a family member that requires and demands adaptation and rebalancing. This stage requires a family to do these things:

- Ask for help. A progressive illness can be exhausting and isolating for the entire family. Hence, it is critically important for the family to move through the enmeshed posture of the acute phase. Families need to seek help and support from extended family and friends during the chronic and terminal stages. Professional care will also be needed in most instances. We will discuss the importance of sharing the responsibility of care with an expanded support system in **Part 4**.

- Communicate effectively. Communication at all levels (within the family, with medical professionals, and with friends) is also critically important during the chronic stage to ensure that neither the patient nor the family feels marginalized or isolated. Both the patient and the family need to be involved with the plan of treatment and care to provide a sense of agency and control.

- Regain control. One of the most debilitating and frustrating elements of a progressive illness is the loss

Speak No Evil

Although my family lived with cancer for eight years, the word "cancer" was rarely spoken in our home! Cancer had historically been a death sentence in my mom's family. There was a reluctance to acknowledge the reality of our situation. If we didn't say "cancer," then perhaps we would be spared. Well, we were not spared. And our inability to talk about our fears and other emotions merely complicated the process for us all. Emotions related to progressive illnesses include fear, guilt, anxiety, frustration, anger, rage, resentment, and hopelessness, to name a few. It is critically important to provide an opportunity to normalize emotions. There is no "right" way to emote; it is dependent on your family's style of communication. The goal is to establish a forum for honest communication that allows for earnest and reflective discussion. How I wish my family had been able to communicate honestly and openly. It would have transformed the experience for all involved.

Uninspired

of control. The body is no longer functioning as expected; the patient is physically or cognitively out of control. Additionally, critical decisions and plans are developed and implemented by a myriad of medical professionals, often with little input from the patient or family. Hence, it is important to maintain a semblance of control over factors within reach.

Express emotions. A family must determine how best to express emotions related to the illness. My family was exceptionally inept regarding effective, heartfelt communication. Reticence to express emotions was reflective of our desire to protect my mom from the reality of the illness. Quite possibly, our unwillingness to discuss the reality of cancer was a behavior of avoidance and denial as well.

Recognize the significance of role changes. During the chronic stage of illness, role changes are needed, often resulting in role reversals (children caring for parents). Some role changes abbreviate or alter life cycles, as in the case with children who assume adult roles and responsibilities. My brother and I were teenagers when our mom was diagnosed with breast cancer. We matured very quickly over the next eight years. Mom and I reversed roles; I was her primary caregiver during the course of her treatment. Additionally,

I took over the responsibility of running the house when Mom was unable to do the typical household chores (cooking, cleaning, laundry, yard work, etc.). To some extent, everyone in the family assumed additional roles. It is no wonder that we all experienced increased levels of stress that manifested in a variety of ways (hypertension, anger, and migraines).

The role changes were equally as difficult for my mom. She felt totally helpless, out of control, and guilty. Although the initial crisis often demands such role changes, redefinition of roles and reassignment of responsibilities is advisable during the chronic stage. Some of the role changes alter the life cycles of individual family members, but this should not be a permanent shift. The roles must be renegotiated and rebalanced at some point to allow the individual to reclaim the appropriate role in the family. Out of necessity, I reversed roles with my mom. However, at some point, I reclaimed the roles of daughter, student, and teenager. The cycle of life continued.

Remission

In some instances (such as cancer), remission is a possibility. Not cure. While in remission, the illness is not progressing or detectable. Although this is fabulous news, it is a stage that necessitates a rebalancing and readjustment of a variety things:

- Roles and responsibilities
- Expectations
- Routines
- Future plans
- Relationships

It is important to realize that a period of remission can generate tremendous anxiety within the family. People become fearful that the next checkup will reveal a recurrence. Any change in health is perceived as a sign that the illness is once again progressing. So the challenge for the family is to live with uncertainty. And the family opportunity is to be present to the moment. A difficult balance to achieve.

Terminal Stage

There is a cultural reluctance in the United States to speak openly about death. We are *scared to death* to talk about the reality of our mortality! However, death is the ultimate change caused by illness. It is part of the lived experience. It is particularly difficult to discuss and accept death when it occurs outside our temporal order (premature death). Our fear of death often leads to an element of secrecy and reluctance to frankly discuss the frightening prognosis.

A terminal illness causes family members to wonder if each special moment will be the last. Throughout the eight years of my mom's illness, every holiday or special occasion was bittersweet as I wondered if it would be the last. Would we share another Christmas? Would Mom be at my wedding? And yet the uncertainty of the future created a sense of urgency, an urgency to appreciate each precious moment. Hence, there was a gift to be discovered in the uncertainty created by cancer. I became intentionally attentive to life and incredibly grateful for the moment.

Although the terminal stage is a very sad and frightening time of life, it is a moment not to be missed. I have listened to far too many people who regret not being present at the death of a family member. Granted, there are situations that preclude our presence (accidental, violent, location, or unexpected deaths). However, if you have the opportunity to prepare and to be present, it is the chance of a lifetime. To prepare for this incredibly sacred time, I would suggest the following:

- Discuss the reality of death.

- Understand the dying process (physical, cognitive, emotional, psychosocial, and spiritual).

- Allow the dying person to talk about hopes and fears.

- Say what you need to say—*do not delay*.

- Express gratitude (give thanks).

- Remember when (life review).

The Invitation to Say Goodbye

The scene is a familiar one. Deserted hallways. The typical sounds of IV pumps and heart monitors. The pungent smell of alcohol and disinfectants. The occasional moan or snore from a patient. You have been a nurse for thirty years, and this is your world.

As you enter room 211, the dim light of a reading lamp reveals a poignant scene. A young woman writes in her journal, curled up on a cot positioned only inches from the hospital bed. Jenny, the daughter of your patient, refuses to leave the bedside of her mother. Over the past five days, Jenny has monitored every breath, every movement, every encounter with the staff. The constant vigil is taking a toll. However, Jenny knows her mother is dying, so she is clinging to every moment. After checking the vital signs and administering needed pain medications, you sit down on the cot with Jenny and ask how she is doing.

Jenny shares her heartbreaking conflict. She wants her mother to live, yet she prays for the suffering to end. This is not an uncommon experience for family members, but Jenny's situation prompts you to share a story, your story. Twenty years ago, you received a call from the emergency room in your home town. An ER physician called to share the tragic news that your mother had died of a heart attack. No signs. No symptoms. No warning. One minute she was puttering in her garden. The next she was dead. Every day for the past twenty years, you have lamented the fact you never had the chance to say goodbye. But tonight is different. Jenny has the opportunity to say what she needs to say. She has the chance to say goodbye. And you are going to make sure she doesn't miss the opportunity of a lifetime. You encourage and invite her to say goodbye to her beloved mother.

Well, I am happy to say that Jenny did accept the invitation. I know this because I am Jenny. The nurse in this story was my vital companion. Her story and encouragement changed my life. I said what I needed to say. I said goodbye. And I am forever grateful.

- Reconcile and forgive (if possible).

- Say "I love you."

- Intentionally say goodbye.

Families often feel tremendous guilt shortly before and immediately after the death of a loved one. It is very difficult to witness the suffering of a loved one. Consequently, we feel conflicted. We don't want our loved ones to die. But we want the suffering to end! Additionally, if the care receiver required extensive care, the family caregivers may experience a sense of relief at the time of death. The journey is finally over. But, wait—that means the person died! This is a very common, understandable reaction. We need not be ashamed. Sometimes, merely normalizing these responses to death is helpful for families.

To Summarize...

- Aging and illness challenge individuals, families, and society. Because we are relational beings, we affect and are affected by the systems in which we live, our families.

- How a family responds to the challenges posed by illness and aging is dependent on key characteristics: family structure and organization, roles and responsibilities, communication, and foundational beliefs.

- Progressive illness poses different challenges at different times. Families must recognize that the different stages require different attitudes, approaches, and responses.

Chapter 5

The Family Legacy of Caregiving

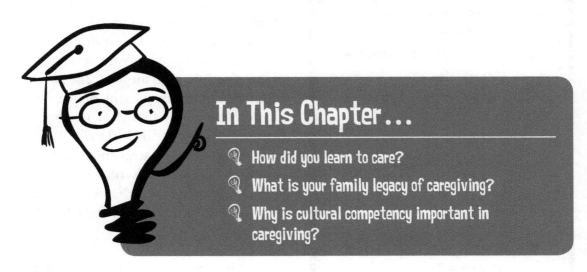

In This Chapter...

- How did you learn to care?
- What is your family legacy of caregiving?
- Why is cultural competency important in caregiving?

I believe most people are inherently compassionate, kind, and caring. However, we learn *how* to care by watching those around us. I had a phenomenal mentor as a child—my mom. She had the heart of a caregiver. Compassion oozed from her pores. By watching my mom serve family, friends, and strangers, I learned how to care for others. My mom sat and listened to our neighbors every morning of the world. She sipped hot tea. Listened intently. Cared unabashedly. Taught me well. Caregiving begins and ends with listening.

We also inherit philosophies of care, the family legacy of caregiving. Family narratives, stories, are passed down from generation to generation. Perhaps

The Family Legacy of Caregiving

What patterns of behavior, attitudes, patterns of communication, and beliefs did you inherit from your family? Which ones serve you well? Which ones do you choose to change?

- Typical caregiver (female, male, eldest child?)
- Roles and responsibilities
- Decision making (who and how?)
- Communication (who and how?)
- Attitudes about death and dying
- Attitudes about illness (what does it mean?)
- Violence and addictive behaviors
- Fears
- Secrets
- Myths
- Spiritual beliefs
- Cultural norms

Perspiration

you never considered the stories told at every family gathering (much to your chagrin) an inheritance. But, they are. Stories are similar to, but essentially different from, the other things inherited from our ancestors. Blue eyes. Big hips. Habits. Preferences. Recipes. Southern drawl. Beliefs. Prejudices. Fears. Hopes. Sense of Humor. Money (maybe). And various and sundry "treasures." The stories convey family attitudes and patterns of behavior related to caregiving. The family narratives reveal the historical who, what, when, where, why, and how of caregiving through the ages. The past certainly informs the present. But we need to acknowledge that historical patterns of care may not serve us well today. We need not accept our caregiving legacies as gospel. Instead, be discriminating. Some stories need to end. Others should be continued, with a little embellishment of course!

Our cultural heritage is also an important factor in how we care for each other. Family narratives reflect cultural norms as well. In order to appreciate the relationship between cultural influences and caregiving, we will first clarify terminology and then explore the topic of cultural competence. This is an important issue for both professional and personal caregivers due to the increased diversity within families and the greater community.

Learn From the Past; Live in the Present

My parents were considered rebels and pioneers in their respective families. My parents were both from Ohio. They met in college. Married. Then moved west of the Mississippi River! Shocking, I know. But it *was* shocking for their families. The family norm was to reside in Ohio, raise your family, work hard, serve the community, and support each other through the trials of life. Pretty simple. Guess my parents were not into simple! As a result, my experience of how a family deals with aging and illness is quite different from that of my parents.

I was born and raised in West Texas. As my great aunt used to say, we lived on the frontier! She refused to visit us for the longest time, fearful that the Wild West was alive and well in Lubbock, Texas. Granted, we had horrific dust storms in the spring. But that is about as wild as it got. In order to stay somewhat connected, we traveled back to Ohio every three years. My mom was afraid to fly, so we hopped the train. It was quite the adventure. My mom made sure that my brother and I had memorable experiences. Exploring the train. Meeting new people. Visiting the Chicago museums and aquarium during our layovers. Fabulous! Once in Ohio, we spent two weeks reconnecting with family.

I always enjoyed our visits to Ohio. But there were times when it was overwhelming. I was accustomed to our small family in Texas. In Ohio, people seemed to come out of the woodwork claiming to be my great aunt, cousin, or whatever! That is usually when my mom would pull me aside and tell me a story. The story served to connect the dots, to connect all the people to me. It was amazing how she could weave everyone into the family tapestry.

As I matured, the nature of the stories matured as well. I heard about the typical family squabbles and conflicts. Remember, all families are fundamentally dysfunctional. But the stories I remember the best dealt with how my mom's family cared for each other. The contrast between her childhood in Ohio and mine in West Texas was stark. My mom had been surrounded by family in Ohio. We had *no* family in Texas. We really *did* live on the frontier! The implications of that geographic isolation were realized many years later when my mom was diagnosed with breast cancer. My family did not have the option of relying on other family members to help with the

On My Way Home

Walking along the streets of her childhood home, my mom pointed out landmarks and shared stories of her life growing up in a quaint Ohio village. I loved listening to the stories and learning more about my mom. She was an extraordinary woman. I savored every moment with her, trying to remember every detail of her stories. Taking mental snapshots of the scenery. Breathing in the summertime fragrances of Ohio. I wanted to remember *everything*. You see, I knew our days were numbered. Although my mom was officially in remission, the constant threat of recurrence was ever present. Knowing I could lose my mom to cancer heightened my appreciation of the moment, and of her stories!

As we passed by a small, unremarkable house, I learned it had been the home of my great-grandparents. So, a remarkable home indeed! We paused for a moment, my mom lost in her memories. A smile crossed her face, and she shared the memories of entering the house through the back door. Without fail, she let the screen door slam, resulting in a reprimand from her grandmother. Yep, my mom the rebel! Evidently, my mom stopped by the house every day after school when her grandfather was ill. Now, I can't even remember what was wrong with him. Guess I didn't remember *all* the details! Anyway, while she was there, her grandmother could run errands, take a nap, or do some other chores. My mom visited with her grandfather, had a snack, and took care of him. I found that to be remarkable. She saw her grandfather *every day*! Unbelievable! But for my mom, her visits happened without a thought, a plan, or a schedule. She reflected, "Of course I stopped by every day. It was on my way home. It's what family did. We cared for each other."

Caring for her family came as naturally as breathing for my mom. She didn't perceive herself as a caregiver to her grandfather. She was merely being a granddaughter! The time afforded her grandmother by her visits wasn't viewed as respite! She was merely being a granddaughter. Yes, a different time. A different place. A different family. A different experience of caring. In that moment, I prayed to hear our screen door slam in Texas if and when my mom's cancer returned. I prayed we would be "on the way home" for our friends. I was going to need the help. I also thought my great-grandmother would get a chuckle out of it. You know what they say about paybacks!

needed caregiving. We did not have the naturally occurring support system of previous generations. Consequently, we relied on each other and our family of choice: our friends. So, although my family legacy of caregiving was informative and useful, it could not be applied as a rigid template of care in Texas. We altered our model of care in light of our available resources and the needs of my mom.

It is important to note that our families and cultural influences inform our ability and willingness to *receive* help as well. Although my mom was the quintessential care*giver*, she found it difficult to be a care *receiver*. This is not an uncommon trait in our society. I often ask those attending my caregiving workshops if they easily ask for or receive help. Not surprisingly, less than 5 percent respond affirmatively. In **Chapter 16**, we will explore our resistance to receiving help in greater detail. But suffice it to say, we learn how to receive care by observing our family as well.

Finally, I want to acknowledge that not all families are loving, kind, and caring. I am well apprised of the severity of dysfunction of some family systems. If this was or is your experience, my heart goes out to you. I will not profess to know how you feel, because I don't. Although my family of origin had its fair share of dysfunction, abuse and violence are thankfully not elements of my family legacy. As I thought about this, I began to wonder how a person learns to care if compassionate care is absent from the family legacy.

I discussed this issue with a dear friend who knows too well the heartache of an abusive family system. This woman is one of the most caring, loving, and generous individuals I have ever known. How did that happen? Well, she offered this perspective. Many of the lessons she should have learned as a child, she learned as an adult. As an adult, she intentionally surrounded herself with kind, caring, and loving people. These mentors taught her how to care for herself and for others. Basically, she courageously chose to end her family legacy of abuse. I am reminded that although we cannot control everything that happens in our lives, we have a choice in how we respond. Be advised, your response could change your life. So choose well. My friend certainly did.

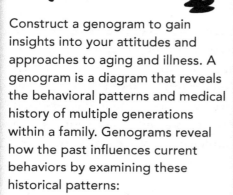

Not Your Basic Family Tree

Construct a genogram to gain insights into your attitudes and approaches to aging and illness. A genogram is a diagram that reveals the behavioral patterns and medical history of multiple generations within a family. Genograms reveal how the past influences current behaviors by examining these historical patterns:

- Family relationships
- Social relationships
- Emotional relationships
- Medical conditions
- Caregiving
- Divorce
- Drug and alcohol abuse
- Physical, sexual, and psychological abuse
- Suicide
- Employment

Perspiration

Tell Me Your Story

A family, when viewed from a historical perspective, often reveals patterns of response, reactions, and attitudes related to aging, illness, and caregiving. As we observe our parents and other family members coping with the challenges of life, we often absorb their attitudes and approaches. We then repeat those same patterns within our own families, thus perpetuating patterns of behavior. Some beneficial. Some detrimental. The good news is that we have the ability to improve the process for future generations.

If previous patterns of behavior and attitudes are not serving you well, do not repeat the mistakes of your elders. Initiate life-giving approaches to companioning the ill and the aging in your family. Create a new legacy! But first you must recognize the patterns.

By examining our family stories, we often discover the historical who, what, when, where, why, and how of caregiving. These elements then generated certain patterns of behaviors and fueled particular attitudes related to caregiving. Our stories reflect individual attitudes, family norms, and cultural influences. I am a very visual person, so I enjoy mapping out various trends within my family. A genogram is a wonderful way to display, or possibly reveal, historical trends and patterns within your family. A *genogram* is a pictorial representation of your family relationships and family history. So, a fancy term for your family tree! But it is so much more. These expanded family trees can be used to trace hereditary tendencies, incidence of disease, caregiving patterns, incidence of addictions, etc. There are computer programs and websites (genopro.com) that facilitate the construction of genograms, making this a useful and accessible tool for individuals and health care providers as well.

My family genogram reveals the prevalence of breast cancer on the maternal side of my family. Since I was a small child, I was told the story of the strong family history of breast cancer. Consequently, breast cancer became an expected part of "my story," a natural extension of my family history. Consequently, I planned accordingly. I believed, without question, that I was doomed to the same fate as my mom and grandmother, death due to breast cancer.

Fifteen years ago, at the invitation of my doctor, I decided to create a new story related to my family's history of breast cancer. The doctor related the facts of my situation in a way I had never considered. He recognized that I was at a higher risk than most women for developing breast cancer. However, the odds were still in my favor. I had a 70 percent chance that I would *never* develop breast cancer! I sat in stunned silence. I had never considered that perspective, because I had been raised to believe I would repeat the pattern I knew all too well. But here was a doctor, an oncologist, telling me that I had the chance to break that deadly pattern! I left that meeting with a new lease on life.

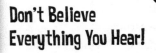

Don't Believe Everything You Hear!

You are not doomed to repeat the mistakes of your ancestors or relive their stories. Write your own narrative. Live *your* life!

IMPORTANT!

I now have a new story, a new life-giving narrative that I choose to embrace. I no longer view myself as an eventual cancer victim. Rather, I am a woman whose family has a strong history of breast cancer; hence, I am being proactive to ensure I remain healthy. The retelling or reconstruction of my narrative does not change the fact that I am at a higher risk than most for breast cancer. However, believing I have the possibility to remain healthy has changed my behavior. Prior to rejecting the notion that I was preordained to develop breast cancer, I literally planned my life assuming I would die at the age of fifty-four, the age my mom died. My resignation to this fate may seem unimaginable to some. Yet I believe it is testament to the power of narrative. Our stories create and generate meaning in our lives in a most powerful way. And the meaning we derive from our stories informs our attitudes and behaviors.

So consider your family stories, your family legacy, carefully. We all have the option and the ability to write our own life-giving narratives. Meaning

Pure Genius!

Different Time, Different Model of Care

"I want my children to see a different way of dealing with this disease. I want my children to know they can and should ask for help!" An amazingly insightful comment from an amazingly courageous man. Josh had been the primary caregiver for his wife since she was diagnosed with Huntington's disease (HD) many years prior to our conversation. HD is a neurodegenerative genetic disorder that affects muscle coordination, impairs cognitive function, and causes psychiatric problems. The journey of HD is long and grueling, often exhausting caregivers. Josh also had four children, all of whom were at risk of developing HD. None had been genetically tested at the time I met Josh. Prior to our meeting, Josh attempted to be all things to all people. However, a recent visit to the ER for extraordinarily high blood pressure convinced Josh that something had to change. He could no longer fly solo. He no longer *wanted* to fly solo. So Josh made the courageous decision to ask his family and friends to help in caring for his beloved wife. He needed to do this for his wife, for himself, and for his children. More than likely, at least one of his children would develop HD. So he wanted his children to see that it was okay to ask for help. In fact, it was more than okay. He wanted that to be the norm. He wanted that to be the family legacy. Josh couldn't reduce the risk of HD for his children. But, perhaps, he could influence how they opted to engage the journey. May it be so.

evolves as individuals and families evolve. We all understand life uniquely; we need not accept life-limiting attitudes and truths from previous generations. Times change. We change. We are wise to critically examine "the stories" passed down to us from previous generations. We can then choose whether to accept or transform our family narratives.

Cultural Competence—A *Must* in Caregiving

The stories of a family reflect historical behaviors and attitudes specific to that family. The narratives also reveal the broader cultural context that significantly impacts approaches to caregiving. Our country and families are becoming increasingly diverse. Hence, we perceive and engage life differently predicated on our family of origin, ethnicity, spiritual beliefs, socioeconomic situation, race, and education. Consequently, each person *sees* life a little differently. We understand illness and aging from slightly different perspectives. And our approaches to caregiving are shaped by our specific cultural expectations and norms. As with family legacies, some cultural expectations serve well within the context of caregiving. Some do not. Adhering strictly to historical, cultural norms can inhibit a family's ability to meet the contemporary demands of caregiving. The challenge then becomes modifying traditional models of care in a respectful manner. This requires that we be culturally competent.

Before proceeding any farther, let's clarify a few terms. First, culture. No, I don't mean the lab experiment growing in your refrigerator! Nope, not referring to your love of opera and caviar. I am talking about everything that makes you *you*! *Culture* is the learned behavior of a group of people that guides practices, decisions, and thought. This learned behavior is transmitted from generation to generation. Culture consists of the following:

- Beliefs
- Symbols
- Thoughts
- Actions
- Customs
- Language

- Institutions
- Life experiences
- Values
- Art
- Folklore
- Traditions

Second, cultural competence. *Cultural competence* is the ability to respectfully and appropriately interact with persons of different cultures. To be culturally competent, you must:

- value diversity (awareness and acceptance of difference);

- appreciate your own cultural perspective (self-awareness);

- comprehend dynamics of difference (awareness of how different cultures interact).

Cultural Competence

Cultural competence is *not* about treating everyone the same, because *we are not*! You must *know* the person in order to serve in culturally appropriate ways.

IMPORTANT!

So why is the issue of culture so important within the context of caregiving? Whether a family member, friend, client, or patient, you must *know* the person in order to serve in a respectful, appropriate manner. If, out of ignorance, you violate a cultural or family norm, you may not be able to regain the respect and trust of the other person. Avoid unintentionally offending another person by taking the time to truly understand the other person. Knowing the person requires more than reading an intake form that notes religious preference, ethnic and racial designations, age, and place of birth. These labels (Episcopalian, Muslim, African American, Texan, etc.) serve as restrictive boundaries, limitations to understanding. Such is the nature of stereotypes. From these initial points of reference, you must then seek to understand by being *respectfully curious*. Ask questions. Express interest. *Listen*! Expand your worldview. Resist the temptation to judge. You are not required to agree with different perspectives. However, every person is worthy of respect and should be honored by the manner in which we serve.

In the introduction, I stressed the importance of being proactive instead of reactive in regard to aging, illness, and caregiving. Now I want to encourage you to be culturally sensitive when developing a plan of care. Sometimes, in our enthusiasm to push the process forward, we assume everyone is on the same page regarding goals, objectives, preferences, and processes. We assume everyone "sees" the situation in the same light. Because of cultural differences, that may not be true. The following list highlights common situations encountered by families dealing with a progressive illness or advanced age. How a family chooses to address the situation is dependent on family and cultural norms:

- Decision making. Who is the decision maker? A critical question when developing a plan of care for an individual. In the United States, we value a person's right to self-determine. However, autonomy is not as highly valued in other cultures. There are alternative models of decision making utilized in other cultures that recognize the physician, the family, or the community as the decision makers. If a decision is needed, you'd better know whom to ask.

- Breaking bad news. Who should be told? In some cultures, it is disrespectful to share bad news with the patient. A terminal diagnosis is to be shared only with the family, not with the patient. In the United States, a patient has the legal right to know. However, the patient may not *want* to know. Before sharing bad news, simply ask the person if he or she wants to know. If not, find out who does.

- Advance directives. We will discuss advance directives extensively in **Chapter 12**. For now, I merely want to highlight the fact that in some cultures, advance directives are distrusted or perceived as unnecessary. You may think advance directives necessary. Others may not.

- Death and dying. It is important to determine if the discussion of death is culturally appropriate. In some cultures, to speak of death is to invite the arrival of death. For others, the discussion of death destroys all hope, a sign of disrespect for the patient. Again, before broaching the subject, determine what is appropriate, sensitive, and respectful.

- Caregiving. Who is expected to care for the aging and the ill in a family? Women? Men? The eldest child? Is it culturally acceptable to ask for assistance outside of the family? In some cultures, to ask nonfamily members to assist with care is shameful. Shameful! For families needing assistance, this is often a cultural expectation that is hard (if not impossible) to overcome. In those instances, you must be culturally sensitive *and* creative.

We Care for Our Own

Many years ago, I was working with an African American family that had some questions about hospice care. As I listened, I realized the family members were exhausted. For the past ten years, they had cared for their mother who suffered from Alzheimer's disease. As we explored the various options for care and assistance, I suggested they consider home health services or perhaps a transition to a memory care unit. Without hesitation, one of the daughters said, "No, thank you. We care for our own." Next?

Example

End-of-life care. Do you want to die at home? Is hospice an option? What is your religious/spiritual tradition? Are plans in place for the desired rituals and services? End of life is a frightening but sacred time. It is also a once-in-a-lifetime opportunity. Cultural competence is critically important in end-of-life care. You don't get a "do-over." So do it right the first time.

Long-term care options. Long-term care outside the home is not an option in some cultures. Family cares for family in the home. When developing a plan of care, this is obviously an important consideration for all involved.

Appropriate touch. As a person ages and becomes ill, by necessity, health care providers must touch the person to provide needed medical care. However, it should be determined if there is a preference for male or female medical professionals. Culturally, it may be inappropriate for a female who is a nonfamily member to touch a male. Before offending, ask!

We are the beneficiaries of those who have gone before us. We inherit attitudes, beliefs, patterns of behaviors, and so much more from our families. Some items are worth keeping. Others prove to be burdensome, mere excess baggage. After reading this chapter, you may realize that your historical family patterns of caregiving no longer serve you well. You may recognize the fear of previous generations hanging on your heart, limiting your ability to live and to love. You may discover your voice and the courage to speak your truth, to write a new narrative. Yes, you may…

To Summarize...

Is caring a consequence of nature or nurture? Both. Human beings are inherently caring. However, we learn to care by observing those around us. So nature *and* nurture are necessary to engage the journey of caregiving. So keep your mind and heart open. There is always something to learn about caring!

Our family legacy of caregiving is reflective of historical attitudes, beliefs, cultural influences, and patterns of behavior. Today, the journey of caregiving is quite different from that of our grandparents. The journey is longer, steeper, and more expensive. And there are fewer hands to help. So we are wise to critically assess historical patterns of care and revise as needed.

We are products of our family and cultural influences. As our society becomes increasingly diverse, it is important to realize that everyone views the journey of illness, aging, and caregiving a bit differently. By seeking to understand the unique perspective of another person, we gain a greater appreciation of the lived experience.

Chapter 6

Long-Distance Caregiving: Bridging the Gap

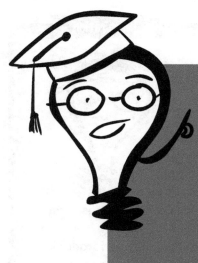

In This Chapter...

- 💡 Why is long-distance caregiving a hot topic today?
- 💡 How can you plan for the unknown?
- 💡 What are the unique challenges of long-distance caregiving?
- 💡 How can technology assist long-distance caregivers?

As we discussed in **Chapter 2**, today's families are quite different from those of previous generations. Today, families are smaller, highly mobile, structurally diverse, and geographically dispersed. Consequently, long-distance caregiving is a common, although challenging, experience for many families in the twenty-first century. Proximity to the care receiver is a critically important factor when developing a plan of care. Based on current demographic trends, long-distance caregiving is here to stay. Hence, we are prudent to prepare well in advance for the long-distance caregiving journey.

The complications associated with long-distance caregiving are numerous, and often frustrating. Quite often, when caring for my family in Texas, I felt as if I were on another planet instead of in another state! Everything seemed *so* much harder. Without feet on the ground, eyes on the issue, and ears tuned to the local station, I struggled to accurately assess situations and respond appropriately. In hindsight (the only time my vision is 20/20), a modicum of preparation would have reduced my level of anxiety tremendously. I don't profess to have all the answers for your specific long-distance caregiving situation. However, by recognizing the unique challenges of long-distance care, you have the opportunity to formulate a tentative plan if and when the occasion arises. Remember, proactive beats reactive every time!

Perspiration

I'll Be There

Remember my friend Kay, from **Chapter 2**? She is the gal who moved back to Wisconsin because that is where she felt "at home." Well, she called a few months ago to discuss some health care concerns. Bottom line, she scheduled a surgery later in the summer at the Mayo Clinic in Rochester, Minnesota. Upon hearing this, I mentally started flipping through my calendar. Kay didn't ask me to be there. But I *wanted* to be there. That's what family does in my world. Before committing to being there, I told Kay I needed to review my calendar. I don't trust my ability to recall all things at the age of fifty-six. I may be forgetful from time to time, but I'm not stupid! I was thrilled to discover that the decks were clear and I could be there for my friend. I immediately called her back and declared, "I'll be there." Typical of Kay, she had already researched my flight options and the shuttle schedule from the airport to the Mayo Clinic. Decisions were made. Details discussed. A plan finalized.

Today, I am happy to report that the surgery went well. I know that Kay appreciated my presence and support. I also know that Kay will be there for me if and when the need arises. She will *want* to be there. That's what family does. A lovely thing indeed.

Advances in communication technology over the past twenty years greatly benefit long-distance caregivers of the twenty-first century. Smartphones, Skype, email, text, and the Internet provide platforms for communication, education, and connection. Regardless of the physical distance between caregiver and care receiver, technology bridges the gap by bringing family, friends, and providers together. Obviously, every person and family will determine how they will utilize the various technological tools and to what extent. It is certainly a resource worthy of consideration.

The Nature of Long-Distance Caregiving

According to the National Institute on Aging, there are over seven million people serving as long-distance caregivers in the United States. What qualifies as long distance? Well, the determination is somewhat arbitrary. For our purposes, if you live more than an hour away from your care receiver, you are a *long-distance caregiver*. Consequently, if you live in a large metroplex, you might be considered a long-distance caregiver based on this definition. I emphasize this point to make sure you recognize yourself as a long-distance caregiver. You may live in the same city as your care receiver. But if you spend an inordinate amount of time en route, please keep reading!

Having previously reviewed the changing demographics in our country as well as the changing nature of families in the twenty-first century, it is obvious why long-distance caregiving is a hot topic. We are an incredibly mobile society. Families rarely reside in the same geographic area. Consequently, when a caregiving need arises, families scramble to cover all the bases. Caregiving is a significant family challenge that is only complicated by geographic dispersion. Consequently, proactive planning is even more important for long-distance caregivers and their care receivers.

How can long-distance caregivers participate in the care of a loved one? Quite often, the geographic separation prohibits frequent visits. So long-distance caregivers must figure out other ways to support the care receiver as well as local family caregivers. Some ideas for consideration include:

- Financial support. Offer to assist with medical expenses. As an illness progresses, the expenses typically increase.

- Emotional support. Contact the care receiver and local family caregivers routinely. Offer support. Listen well.

A Walk Interrupted

As I considered my approach shot to the ninth green, I noticed a golf cart advancing at a high rate of speed. The driver of the cart was waving frantically and yelling my name! I was home for a long weekend, visiting my dad, and enjoying a round of golf. So this intrusion was quite unexpected, and actually unwelcome. As it turned out, my godmother was in the ER of a local hospital having suffered a ministroke. I needed to get there as quickly as possible.

As you might imagine, I was distraught! My godmother, Aunt Jane, was like a second mother to me. She meant the world to me! Driving to the hospital, I tried to put a lid on my emotions. I needed a plan! You see, my godmother lived alone. She didn't have children. And, I was planning to return to Colorado the next day. *Not!* Okay. Plan B. There *is* a Plan B, right?

Uninspired

Daily contact. Send emails or text on a daily basis. Caregivers and care receivers often feel isolated. A one-line text serves as an important connection to the outside world.

Respite for local caregivers. Local caregivers need breaks, extended breaks. Offer to fill in as caregiver for one to two weeks.

Online assistance. Knowledge is power when it comes to caregiving, illness, and aging. Long-distance caregivers can gather a tremendous amount of information via the Internet regarding resources, Medicare and Medicaid, medications, health insurance, online bill paying, etc.

Facilitate communication. Long-distance caregivers can provide regular updates to family and friends regarding the status of the care receiver.

Caregiving, local or long distance, is an emotional roller coaster. One moment you are cruising along, enjoying life. The next, you are screaming downhill into a dark, deep pit wondering what went wrong! In **Part 3**, we will discuss the issue of caregiver stress and how to manage these emotional highs and lows. However, guilt is an emotion that is particularly problematic for long-distance caregivers and therefore warrants further discussion.

Long-distance caregivers often feel guilty because of their physical absence. They weren't there for the medical emergency. They didn't recognize the initial signs of an illness. They aren't there to help with the house, the yard, and the chores. They aren't there to provide emotional support. They aren't at the bedside. But they are concerned. They do care. They are afraid. They want to help. And . . . they feel guilty.

Example

Break My Heart

I was fortunate that Aunt Jane, my godmother, made the decision to sell her house and move to a long-term care community. I didn't have to tell her to sell the house. Not that she would have listened to me anyway! She was wise enough to realize after a series of ministrokes, it was no longer wise to live alone. This was a courageous decision on her part. She sold the home that she and my godfather built and shared for over thirty years. A lifetime of memories. A sense of belonging. Regardless, the reality was apparent. It was no longer safe for her to live there.

Moving from her home to a small apartment in a long-term care community required planning and the assistance of many. I recall my brother struggling to get Aunt Jane's refrigerator through the doorway of her apartment, ultimately removing the door. I remember my sister-in-law doing countless things to move the process along. And I remember the first night Aunt Jane stayed in her apartment, alone. After all the "to dos" had been accomplished. After we enjoyed a lovely meal. The reality came home to roost. Aunt Jane was not going home, at least not to the home we had all known and loved for so many years.

For the rest of her life, I would have to imagine her in an unfamiliar, one-bedroom apartment instead of the home I knew so well. But I would not have to imagine the intensity of her pain or the depth of her sorrow, because I heard it. After saying goodbye and hugging her, the door closed. In the privacy and silence of her apartment, she could no longer mute her grief. She sobbed uncontrollably. And so did I. The sound of a broken heart is unlike any other. It haunts me to this day.

Long-distance caregivers must accept the reality of the situation. Recognize limitations. Identify possibilities (ways to support the caregiving process from a distance). Additionally, local family caregivers must appreciate the limitations of the long-distance caregivers and collaboratively discuss the possibilities. In the section on planning, we will discuss the importance of assigning roles and responsibilities such that certain family members do not feel overly burdened. When local family caregivers feel resentful, they often enhance a long-distance caregiver's sense of guilt. It's all about balance and shared responsibilities.

As noted in the introduction, caregiving is about care *giving* and care *receiving*. Therefore, we need to consider the issue of long-distance caregiving from the *giver's* perspective as well as from the *receiver's* perspective. Many care receivers feel as if they are burdens on their families—physically, emotionally, and financially. To witness long-distance family members incurring travel expenses, taking time off from work, and being separated from their own families serves to intensify the care receiver's sense of guilt. So, needless to say, there is more than enough guilt to go around! Guilt serves no one well. Instead, families benefit from honest, compassionate conversations between caregivers and the care receiver. Air out your emotions, frustrations, and concerns. More often than not, you will find common ground (I hope!). From there, collaboratively create a plan of care.

Plan, Plan, Plan

I *love* a good plan! In fact, I actually enjoy developing plans. Consequently, I think planning is underrated and unjustly disparaged. There was a time in my life (corporate years) when I actually carried around a five-year planner. I agree, somewhat reluctantly, that was a bit over the top. But it served a purpose. As I considered the next five years, I had to anticipate needs, project growth, and identify resources. Since I am not clairvoyant, my plans were subject to adjustments and refinement as conditions changed. It was a work in progress. But the plan served as a stable foundation from which to make course corrections.

The same is true when developing a plan for long-distance caregiving. There is *no* way you can anticipate everything that could possibly happen. Too many variables. But that does not preclude the consideration of possible scenarios. If long-distance caregiving is on the horizon (or at your front door), proactive planning will save you time, energy, and anxiety. Some aspects of the plan will not be implemented until the caregiving need arises. But anticipation of the process prepares you to hit the ground running. To meet the challenge of long-distance caregiving, you will need to do these things:

- Convene a family meeting to coordinate care.

- Identify local and long-distance caregivers (family and friends).

- Determine who will serve as the primary caregiver.

- Discuss roles and responsibilities.

- Organize legal, financial, and medical documents.

- Discuss and finalize advance directives.

- Leverage the strengths of family members.

- Establish goals of care.

- Identify wants and needs; discuss hopes and fears.

- Include the care receiver in developing the plan of care.

- Establish a system of communication; provide status updates to family and friends.

- Meet with medical staff and schedule regular updates.

- Understand the disease process and prognosis.

- Anticipate needs predicated on prognosis and expected disease trajectory.

- Identify local resources.

- Identify sources of financial assistance.

- Identify future housing needs and anticipate any needed transitions.

- Periodically revisit the plan.

- Coordinate personal caregiving with professional services.

- Know your limits as a long-distance caregiver.

- Plan for the additional expense of long-distance caregiving.

- Arrange time off from work (vacation, family leave, etc.).

- Schedule quality time to *be* with the care receiver.

Uninspired

Perhaps You Should Ask!

Following our dad's stroke, we (my brother Richard, his wife Dana, and I) had to make some important decisions. At the time, our dad lived alone. After the stroke, living alone was not advisable. So we explored various options and finally located a condo not far from one of his friends. Thinking this a fabulous solution, we made plans to move in short order. As luck would have it, there was an ice storm in West Texas the weekend of the move. However, we are hearty stock and pushed through the inclement weather. After an incredibly *long* weekend, we rejoiced in a job well done!

Turns out, we were much happier about the move than our dad. We failed to recognize that our dad was afraid to live alone after his stroke. Consequently, he *never* spent a night in the condo we so carefully appointed and prepared. Instead, he moved in with a friend who agreed to care for him.

Note to self. *Ask* the person what is wanted and needed. Odds are, the person will tell you! This will save you a lot of time, energy, and frustration. Hopefully, you'll miss the joy of moving a household in an ice storm. That was an experience I could have lived without!

Long-Distance Challenges

When you don't have feet on the ground and eyes on your loved ones, it is hard to know what is actually going on. It's amazing how "together" a person can sound on the phone for a short conversation when in reality the person's life is falling apart. So, words to the wise. Listen well. Trust your gut. Anticipate what could happen. If possible, see for yourself.

Hidden Truths

Long-distance caregiving poses some unique challenges. Because of the geographic separation, long-distance caregivers cannot easily assess the situation. Consequently, they often rely on the care receiver, other family members, friends, or medical professionals for status updates. As you know, some sources are more reliable than others. Sometimes, long-distance caregivers just need to *see* what is going on. But it's often hard to decide *when* to go. With job responsibilities, travel expenses, and personal relationships, long-distance caregivers must be prudent about scheduling visits. Yet, seeing is believing. Observing the situation firsthand often reveals information that has been withheld for far too long. Care receivers frequently attempt to protect loved ones from the reality of the situation. But in order to provide adequate and compassionate care, families must know the truth about the situation.

Undetected Elder Abuse

Elder abuse is an important issue for local and long-distance caregivers. However, in the case of long-distance caregivers, the challenge is detection and/or recognition of abuse. Without feet on the ground, abuse can go undetected for far too long. Long-distance caregivers need to be attentive for any indication of abuse, whether at the hands of a family or professional caregiver or within an institutional setting. If there is cause for concern, there are organizations, such as Adult Protective Services, to assist in addressing and resolving the issue. An unannounced visit by the long-distance caregivers can be quite revealing as well. Listen to your gut. If you think something is wrong, check it out.

What Happened?

At an Alzheimer's Association conference several years ago, I met a woman whose mother had the disease. Mona shared that she and her siblings had recently assumed the responsibility of care for their mother. They were all attending the conference to gain a better understanding of what to expect in the years to come. The diagnosis had been a shock, and they felt totally unprepared. As Mona shared her story, I sensed an overwhelming sense of guilt and regret as well.

Mona and her siblings lived out of state. None had been home for a visit in over two years. She made no excuses. Merely stated the facts. During that time, she faithfully called her mother every Sunday afternoon to check in. Never once did she suspect something was going on. Her mother sounded strong, happy, and in control. Today, she wondered how she could have been so oblivious to the profound changes in her mother.

Two months ago, Mona and her siblings decided to come home for a long-overdue reunion. Upon arrival, they knew something was terribly wrong. Their mother had always maintained a well-organized, spotless home. But that day, dishes filled the sink. Stacks of mail littered the dining room table. The kitchen smelled of mold and spoiled food. Mona and her siblings were speechless. What happened? Their mother stood calmly in the middle of this heartbreaking scene, seemingly unaware of her children's distress. Mona had no idea how to respond to "welcome home."

Mona's mother did what so many of us do when confronted with a dire reality. She denied it. She hid it. However, with a progressive dementia, the reality cannot be denied indefinitely. Mona and her siblings felt guilt and remorse for missing the signs of dementia. "We should have known." Well, it's hard to "know" if you aren't there.

It is also quite possible that Mona's mother was not in denial. Instead, she chose to protect her children from the reality of dementia. This is a very common scenario. We attempt to protect those we love by hiding the harbingers of illness and death. Although the intent is noble, hiding the truth is often hurtful. Precious time is lost to plan and to accept the reality of the situation. So, do not delay. We can't protect our loved ones from the realities of life. But, we can invite them to walk with us to the end of the road. A sacred journey indeed.

Local and Long-Distance Caregiver Conflict

Over the past decade, I have conducted numerous programs on caregiving. At every program, at least one person complains about an out-of-state sibling who doesn't "get" how hard it is to care for an aging parent. The proximal child deals with the issues of caregiving on a daily basis. The distant child flies in once a year to "check on Mom." More often than not, tempers flare, accusations fly, and relationships can be forever damaged. This particular scenario highlights the need to plan well. Families must establish the ground rules of care early in the process. Roles and responsibilities. Plan of care. Etc. Without that thoughtful discussion and planning process, the journey is usually much more difficult and potentially contentious.

The Move

The complicating factor of long-distance caregiving is obvious. Long distance! So if we can eliminate the factor of long distance, we're home free, right? Not so fast. Regardless of who moves, relocation is very disruptive. Remember our discussion of family systems and how we are all interconnected? Well, a relocation of the caregiver *or* the care receiver sends shock waves throughout the system. For the aging and/or ill person, a transition to a new "home" is particularly problematic. In many cases, the transition is recognized in hindsight by the family as the beginning of the end.

Take Advantage of Technology

The Internet and social media have long been recognized as tremendous tools for networking, educating, and creating online communities. This technology is proving to be a valuable and needed resource for local and long-distance caregivers as well as care receivers. The realized value of social media is dependent on personal preference, technological savvy, and imaginative integration of technology. However, for individual and families who choose to leverage this powerful platform, it can absolutely change the experience of caregiving.

Many caregivers and care receivers feel isolated. Illness and aging result in physical and/or cognitive impairments, often limiting the mobility

I Want to Go Home!

Peggy looked out her condo window at the lush gardens. Spring in Atlanta was truly an amazing season. This morning, the cardinals serenaded her while the squirrels entertained her with acrobatic moves worthy of the Cirque du Soleil. Sounds lovely, right? For some, perhaps. But not for Peggy. She just wanted to go home.

Last year, Peggy moved to Atlanta to be closer to her daughter. It had become increasingly difficult for her daughter to travel to Seattle for Peggy's occasional medical issues. And Peggy realized she wasn't getting any younger and would eventually need more help. So when her daughter suggested she move, Peggy thought it a good idea.

Now, a year later, Peggy was desperately lonely and homesick. She missed her routine of walking to the market every day and visiting with her friends along the way. There were so many things to miss. Church. Book club. Bridge club. Her favorite bookstore. And, of course, all her friends.

Granted, the move made life easier for her daughter. No more long trips away from the family. Fewer travel expenses. Less time off from work. All of that was fabulous for her daughter and her family. But what about Peggy? Yes, she was closer to family. But, shortly after settling in, it became apparent the family had little time to spend with her. With three teenagers, a husband, and her job, Peggy's daughter was always on the run. Not surprising, yet disappointing.

Peggy should have known the move would be hard. At eighty-five, it's hard to start over in a strange place. You can't replace lifelong friends who know you from the inside out. However, her daughter had been quite persuasive. Gorgeous condo. Great community. Family close by. It seemed like a good idea. But today, Peggy regretted the decision. She resented her daughter for moving her cross-country only to be ignored. Today, Peggy wanted nothing more than to go home.

Peggy's story is a common one. Families struggling to care for a loved one long distance often deem relocation to be the best option. Best for whom? The long-distance caregivers? The care receiver? We must understand the motivation for relocation and the implications for all involved. Leaving a beloved home and community is difficult. It is a tremendous loss, a loss that must be acknowledged and mourned. As we age, relocation can be destabilizing and isolating. So, before choosing to move, carefully consider all options. Remember, there is no place like home.

of an individual. Sometimes it is just too hard to get out and about. However, technology serves as the conduit to connect with other people, entertainment, information, and community. Technology can hook you up! Smartphones, computers, email, texting, Skype, and Facebook are just a few of the ways to stay connected with family and friends. It is also an efficient and effective way to update family and friends on the status of a care receiver.

If you don't have access to a computer, check around. Public libraries usually have computers for public use. If you live in a long-term care community, check to see if there is a computer room for residents. And, if you lack computer skills, sign up for a class. Staying connected to your family, friends, and online communities (that you will join) can be life giving, if not life sustaining.

One final note about technology and caregiving. The Internet is a powerful planning tool for families dealing with aging and illness. Needed information to develop a plan of care is at your fingertips. In **Part 4**, you will discover how the Internet can assist in creating a community of care to share in the responsibilities of caregiving. A good thing indeed! If you have been critical of technology to this point, hang on. I am going to do my best to woo you over. You'll be texting, tweeting, and Skyping before you know it!

To Summarize...

- Long-distance caregiving is quite common in the United States today due to the changing nature of families and increased life expectancy. Caregiving is usually hard enough. Long distances complicate caregiving.

- Long-distance caregiving shouldn't come as a surprise if your family is geographically dispersed. However, families appear shocked and amazed more often than not. To avoid a frantic cross-country scramble, plan in advance.

- Long-distance caregiving, by its nature, creates unique challenges for families. The more common complications include incomplete or inaccurate information, undetected elder abuse, internal family conflicts, and ill-advised moves.

- Technology facilitates and supports the long-distance caregiving process. Access to information, family, friends, entertainment, and the greater community mitigates the sense of isolation so often experienced by caregivers and care receivers.

Chapter 7

Critter Care

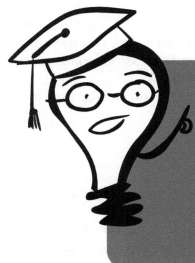

In This Chapter...

- What is the magical connection between humans and animals?
- What do animals have to teach us about caregiving?
- How are we called to care for our critters?
- Who will care for our critters when we can't?

I love critters. Always have. Always will. My family of choice includes cats and dogs, always. I am not alone in my love of critters. According to American Pet Products Association, over 60 percent of all households in the United States have a pet. Boomers love critters! Consequently, over 60 percent of households will be called to care for aging and ill critters. Caring for critters is not unlike caring for humans. In fact, the similarities are fascinating—physically, emotionally, financially, and spiritually. So, repeat after me. *Prepare to care*! Our critters are worth it.

Critters, particularly dogs, typify the concept of caregiving perfectly. First, critters serve as incredible caregivers. I have yet to meet a human caregiver who is as masterful as a dog in regard to presence, nonverbal communication, and unconditional love. We have much to learn from our canine friends about caregiving. On the flip side, critters graciously receive our help and ultimately embrace the reality of death. Lessons we would be wise to learn, sooner rather than later.

I have cared for humans and critters. Family and clients. Friends and strangers. The old and the young. Each journey of caregiving requires different things of me. And with each journey, I receive different blessings in return. My cats and dogs have been incredible mentors over the past twenty years. It has been the journey with my critters that I find the most poignant. Perhaps it is because I feel a heightened sense of responsibility to "speak" for my critters. Whatever. When caring for my critters, I feel raw and exposed. The journey begins the moment our eyes meet and our hearts connect. The journey ends when their eyes close and my heart breaks. We can prepare in advance for some aspects of care. We can't adequately prepare for a broken heart. So we do the best we can.

The Human-Animal Bond

Historically, animals served in a variety of roles that enhanced the quality of life of human beings. Animals provided (and continue to provide) protection, companionship, labor, sport, healing, and guidance. In fact, the human-animal bond appears to be quite ancient indeed and not restricted to a physical relationship. In ancient Greece, Asklepios, the god of medicine, used sacred dogs to heal the blind. Even in Zoroastrian Persia, it was believed that the gaze of a dog could release a person's soul into the afterlife. Thus, animals have historically served to meet the physical, emotional, and spiritual needs of humans. Fascinating, but not surprising at all. For those of us who love our critters, we *know* the incredible bond between humans and animals. Often the bond defies explanation, but the bond exists nonetheless.

The National Love Affair with Critters

We are a critter-loving country! Check out the Humane Society of the United States (humanesociety.org) or the American Pet Products Association (americanpetproducts.org) to discover some amazing statistics about critters in our country. The trend in human families may be toward fewer

I am sooo happy!

Several years ago, I visited an equine therapy center. I wanted to understand the therapeutic benefits of equine therapy by observing the process. At this particular facility, people with a variety of needs benefited in extraordinary ways. As is often the case, a large percentage of the clients were children diagnosed with autism. There was one little guy who grabbed my heart that day. Ryan was a precious four-year-old. Curly blond hair. Gorgeous blue eyes. Cherubic cheeks. Severely autistic.

I learned from his therapist and parents that Ryan rarely uttered a sound. However, I could tell that he loved riding "his" horse. Murphy was a fine steed. And Ryan sat tall in the saddle. Ryan and Murphy obviously shared a special bond. Thus, the riding class was the highlight of Ryan's week, according to his parents.

The day I visited the equine center happened to be the first day of the summer session. The horses had been "on break" the previous two weeks, enjoying a much-needed rest after eight weeks of riding classes. As you might imagine, the children were eager to reunite with their horses that first day. Ryan ran into the equine center, obviously excited to get on "his" horse. Once he was settled in the saddle, Murphy was led around the arena by trained volunteers. It wasn't long before I heard someone giggling. At first, I thought it was one of the volunteers. But the sound was that of a child. As I glanced around the arena, I saw Ryan grinning from ear to ear, giggling uncontrollably! He then looked directly at me and said, "I am sooo happy!"

Those were the first words spoken by Ryan during his riding sessions. Everyone in the arena that morning experienced a miracle. As I witnessed the sheer joy of a child, tears streaming down my face, I silently thanked Murphy for touching the heart of this precious child in ways we could not. A miracle indeed. And, yes, I was sooo happy!

children, but the increasing prevalence of critters (all varieties) bucks that demographic trend. Please note, my experience is predominantly with dogs, cats, and horses. I realize you may prefer rabbits, ferrets, or birds. So when I refer to critters, think of *your* critter of choice. With that said, I would like to share a bit of data to reinforce the importance of this issue of critter care in the United States:

- Sixty percent of households have a critter.

- Thirty percent of households have at least one dog.

- Thirty-three percent of households have at least one cat.

If you do not own a cat or dog, our household has you covered! We are well above the average. That means we incur significant expense just for the basics. We also assume the risk of additional medical costs as our critters age or become ill. Our household is not unique. In 2013, the estimated bill for critter care is:

- $21.2 billion for food;

- $4.5 billion for grooming and boarding services;

- $13.2 billion for supplies and over-the-counter medications;

- $14.2 billion for vet care.

This is not chump change! Total expenditures for 2013 will approach $53 *billion*. We invest in the basic care of our critters (food, supplies, grooming, and boarding). But we also invest in acute/terminal care/end-of-life care, amounting to over $14 billion. If you have ever had a pet in critical or acute care, you know how quickly expenses accumulate. Hence, the need for a plan of care for your critter is apparent. Prior to a health care crisis, you need to seriously consider what you would want to do, what you can afford to do, and what you should do. Not easy questions to answer in the midst of a crisis with your critter. Believe me, I know.

Return on Investment

The human-animal bond benefits people physiologically, psychologically, emotionally, and spiritually. So, when analyzing the return on investment, critters appear to be a wise investment, at least from my perspective. It is well documented by scientific research and anecdotal studies that critters:

- lower blood pressure;
- reduce stress;
- lessen risk of heart disease;
- lower health care costs;
- lessen depression;
- provide meaningful companionship;
- offer affection (unconditional love);
- symbolize a spiritual presence.

Just in case you needed one more reason to get that sweet kitten, puppy, or rabbit, there you go!

Critters as Caregivers

Critters are intuitive caregivers. We don't have to say a word, do we? Our critters just "know" when we are ill or are feeling blue. In fact, animals can often anticipate a health care crisis. Many people rely on specially trained animals to warn of seizures or heart attacks. In hospice, it is well known that animals sense when death is imminent. And in the case of posttraumatic stress disorder, specifically trained dogs enable veterans to reengage with life. Every day, there are stories of how critters enrich our lives and enable us to live happier and healthier lives. They are *the* best caregivers in the world.

I have experienced the healing power of critters personally as well as professionally. As a chaplain intern in hospice, I witnessed the "miracle" of therapy animals with the dying and the bereaved. Consequently, I was inspired to learn more! To augment my seminary training, I took numerous classes related to animal-assisted therapy. As a result, I have a greater appreciation for how and why critters facilitate healing where humans seemingly fail. Service dogs and therapy animals serve humans in amazing ways, enabling humans to navigate life physically, emotionally, and spiritually. Critters understand the power of presence and possess an innate ability to connect at the heart-and-soul level. If we are wise enough to observe our critters and service animals in action, we will learn the sacred art of giving and receiving care. A blessing indeed.

Healers and Guides

Critters are gifted healers and guides. Unlike humans, who tend to compartmentalize types of treatments, critters serve as a holistic balm offering healing for the mind, body, and spirit. How does the presence of a dog lower a person's blood pressure? Why does someone with Alzheimer's disease become less anxious and less aggressive when a dog is present? No doubt, these are questions that will be bandied about for years to come. Perhaps the healing derived from interacting with critters is due to our experience of being heard, being honored, being loved, and being accepted without judgment. I don't always need a rational explanation for what I observe or experience. Instead, I choose to accept the mystery and embrace the blessings.

Masters of Nonverbal Communication

Critters are wonderful instructors in the art of nonverbal communication. Although critters can communicate verbally (i.e., barking, growling, etc.), nonverbal messages are more common and very effective. Body posture, facial expressions, and ear position (referred to as "social signaling") are a few ways in which critters express emotions and convey information to other animals and humans. Not only do the critters project nonverbal signals, but they receive and interpret them as well. Our critters read us like an open book. So, if you want to fly under the radar screen, you'd better steer clear of your critters. You can run, but you can't hide!

Consequently, by observing the interaction of critters with other people, we can gain new insights into what people are feeling but are unable to express verbally. Within our families or in a clinical setting, critters can signal who is in need of care. They can point us in the right direction. Critters hear what is not said, sense pain that is not known, and provide healing that is transformative. So pay attention. We have much to learn. Stop, look, and listen.

The Power of Presence

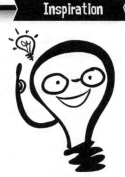

Growing up, I was not familiar with the journey of dementia. My family legacy was that of cancer. However, I learned of the journey of Alzheimer's disease by companioning families, listening, and observing. Interestingly enough, I learned the importance of presence by observing the interaction between a remarkable dog and a person with Alzheimer's disease.

Ron was a resident in a memory care unit. His condition had deteriorated rapidly over the past few weeks. Previously mobile, communicative, and fairly cooperative, Ron was now confined to a wheelchair, shouted profanities, and was physically aggressive toward staff and other residents. The staff employed a variety of approaches and interventions, without success. Ron was described as "tormented." At the suggestion of the unit's social worker, a therapy dog was scheduled to visit Ron. Gretchen was a black lab, an exceptional therapy dog. Ron needed exceptional.

I just happened to be in the memory unit visiting a friend's father the day Gretchen met Ron. When Gretchen entered the memory care unit, you could feel the energy change. Dogs have that effect on people! Many of the residents and staff came over to greet Gretchen. Slowly, Gretchen and her handler made their way over to Ron. He was seated in a chair that had a tray, thus restricting his ability to stand. I could see his anxiety level rise as the dog and handler approached. He felt threatened. The handler recognized this as well and opted to turn things over to Gretchen.

When Ron started screaming and swinging his arms, Gretchen stopped and sat down. She didn't look directly at Ron, but she closely monitored his activity. As Ron calmed down, Gretchen inched her way slowly across the room. With every advance, she stopped to assess Ron's reaction. It took Gretchen about ten minutes to make her way over to Ron. She positioned herself such that Ron couldn't kick her, but he could pet her if so inclined.

As Gretchen sat patiently beside Ron, he physically changed. His shoulders relaxed. His face softened. His eyes filled with tears. And then, he slowly reached out to Gretchen, gently touching her soft muzzle. Gretchen rewarded his kindness by tenderly licking the palm of his hand. And Ron smiled. He was no longer tormented. Because Gretchen had the courage to be present to his pain, Ron no longer felt alone. Such is the power of presence.

Critters Caring for Critters

If you have more than one critter in your family, I am sure you have witnessed your critters caring for each other. It matters not if you have the same species. Critters are evidently culturally competent as well as intuitive! All are welcome and all are honored. I have witnessed this caring interaction countless times, and I always marvel at a critter's intuitive response to care for those in need.

Several years ago, JoAnne (you met her in **Chapter 2**, my best friend and housemate) and I rescued five kittens found in a ditch. At the time, we had one dog, Kemah. Kemah was a gorgeous Samoyed/Great Pyrenees mix that I rescued when living in Texas. He was an amazing dog indeed! Imagine Kemah's surprise when we walked in the door with five meowing kittens! Not surprisingly, Kemah ended up raising the three kittens we kept. Today, our cats project the same loving, compassionate spirit as Kemah. Family legacies of caregiving are not restricted to the human species!

Critters as Care Receivers

In the fall of 2012, our beloved dog, Bella, developed a very rare autoimmune disorder. Our sweet Australian shepherd/cattle dog was only five years old. Shocked doesn't begin to describe our reaction! We were completely blindsided. If untreated, she would die within days or possibly weeks of diagnosis. If treated, she had only a fifty-fifty chance of survival. It was our journey with Bella that prompted a chapter on critter care in this book.

Bella spent a week in acute care following her diagnosis. So JoAnne and I also spent a week in acute care! The staff was incredibly kind. We were allowed to stay with Bella the majority of the time. I know it must have made their jobs harder having us literally underfoot. I will be forever grateful for having the opportunity to companion Bella through the early stages of treatment. It meant so much to all of us.

The day Bella received a blood transfusion, I set up camp in her four-by-eight-foot concrete kennel. There was just barely enough room for both of us. I had one hand on my computer and one hand on Bella. Interestingly enough, I wrote the proposal for this book as I sat with Bella. Needless to say, she served as my writing muse and continues to do so today.

No Words Required

I have always appreciated the importance of listening. In fact, I consider myself a fairly accomplished listener. However, a visit to a children's grief center taught me the importance of hearing what is *not* said.

The day I visited the center, I observed a class of children twelve to eighteen years of age. The children had all experienced a significant loss. There was a trained adult paired with each child. During the session, the adult served as a mirror for the child, repeating words and mimicking behaviors. A technique commonly used in children's grief centers throughout the United States.

Abby, a thirteen-year-old who had been attending sessions at the center for the past year, captured my attention. She was a rather quiet, reserved child who chose to express her grief through artistic expression rather than actions or words.

There was also a special guest scheduled for the class that day. Radar, a golden retriever, was a well-known therapy dog in the community. Without fail, Radar could "sniff out" the child who needed him most. He could detect the unspoken, hidden pain within a grieving child. Without question, Radar lived up to his name!

As the session began, Radar checked in with everyone in the room. He approached every child, wagging his tail and offering a gentle nudge here and there. This touch-and-go behavior occurred repeatedly throughout the session, but Radar always ended up sitting or standing by Abby. If Abby moved, Radar followed. It was a lovely, spontaneous dance as Radar followed Abby's lead.

The session was structured, with the exception of the final ten minutes. At the end of the session, the children had the option to choose an activity. Abby chose to lie on the floor and gaze at the ceiling mural. Radar stretched out beside her, laying his head upon her chest. Gradually, the dog and the girl began breathing as one. Radar was literally breathing life back into this young girl! Abby relaxed as Radar continued to look lovingly at her. Slowly, a smile graced Abby's face. She was at peace, if only for a moment.

As I observed this sacred moment, I knew I was seeing more than a young girl snuggling with a dog. I witnessed a spiritual presence that embraced, loved, and healed a wounded child. Without words, Radar sensed Abby's pain. Without words, Radar initiated the healing process. Stop. Look. *Listen.*

Over the course of two months, Bella taught me so much about the caregiving journey. I always thought Bella a wise soul. And I was right. In the midst of her struggle to live, she demonstrated courage, determination, grace, gratitude, and ultimately acceptance. Bella died on November 17, 2012. But our memories of her are very much alive. My hope is that by sharing what I witnessed and learned from Bella, you and your family will be better prepared to care for your beloved critter.

Intensity of Care

After Bella was diagnosed with a life-threatening condition, our lives were not our own. The demands of caregiving were all consuming. You should know that JoAnne and I make a formidable team when it comes to caregiving. But we were not prepared for this journey with Bella. The intensity of care Bella required matched or exceeded any of our previous caregiving experiences. So please do not underestimate the daunting challenges of critter care, such as the ones we experienced with Bella:

- Medical emergency. We were totally unprepared. We had no pet insurance.

- Lack of knowledge about the disease process. We had never heard of this condition before. We had to assimilate a tremendous amount of information in a compressed period of time. Decisions had to be made.

- Juggling schedules. JoAnne and I both work. When Bella was discharged from the animal hospital, one of us had to be home with her. We managed to cover the bases, but it was challenging!

- Incontinence. Due to the condition or the medications, Bella became incontinent. As with people, this complicated the caregiving process.

- Special diet. We went through at least ten different brands of food trying to get Bella to eat.

- Adverse drug reactions. Incontinence, stomach issues, and muscle wasting were a few of the more concerning side effects of the drugs.

- Administering drugs. Bella was on so many drugs when she finally came home that we created a schedule. I set alarms throughout the house so we didn't miss a scheduled dose.

- Physical changes. Due to muscle wasting, Bella became weak and no longer enjoyed long walks. I bought stairs to assist her in getting up and down from my bed.

- Mental changes. Bella lost her *zest* for life toward the end of life. Depressed? Quite possibly.

- Blood transfusions. Did you know there is a blood bank specific to dogs? Also, there are services that provide dog blood donors. Who knew?

- Changes in sleep habits. Bella didn't sleep more than two hours at a time. She constantly needed to go outside to urinate. Needless to say, I couldn't sleep longer than two hours at a time either!

- Disease progression. As Bella's condition worsened, symptom management was a constant challenge.

- Financial concerns. You can say it is not about the money, but in reality, the expenses are a *huge* concern unless you have unlimited resources. In two months, we spent over $5,000. Know this going in. Be prepared.

- Not knowing. Bella could not articulate her wishes at any point in her journey. Yes, we looked for signs. We prayed for guidance. We sought wise counsel. But ultimately, the decisions were ours.

- Option of euthanasia. Having companioned patients and families at the end of life, I have heard numerous people lament the fact that euthanasia is not an option for people. This is not meant to be a forum for debate regarding the issue of euthanasia. But I will say this, having the option of euthanasia for our critters is a tremendous responsibility indeed. It is one of the hardest decisions we have to make for the critters we love so dearly. With Bella, the option proved to be blessing and burden.

Gracious Receivers of Care

I was blessed to know and love Bella for a little over five years. In that time, I learned so much from my dear friend. But no greater lesson was offered than that of being a gracious care receiver. In the last two months of her life,

Bella allowed us to completely care for her. We saw her at her worst and her best. And everything in between. She remained loving, open, vulnerable, and incredibly grateful for all she received. And because there was no resistance on her part, we were allowed to walk with her, every step of the way. It was one of the hardest journeys of my life, and one of the most meaningful. Bella's willingness to receive made all the difference. I hope to emulate Bella's courageous and gracious attitude at my journey's end.

Is It Time?

Critters exhibit an inherent understanding of the life cycle. We are born, and we die. In between, life presents challenges as well as opportunities. We can't control everything that happens in life, but we do retain control of our responses. Critters are naturally present in the moment. Not mired in the past or lost in speculation about the future. Critters are present to the here and now. And because of that, they seem to know when it is time, time to move on. Our challenge is to read the signs.

In the past year, we have said goodbye to Bella and one of our cats, Whisper. Each time, we struggled in knowing when it was time to say goodbye. And each time, our critter let us know. Oh that humans could be that tuned into the rhythms of life!

Necessary Critter Plans

Our intense caregiving journey with Bella the fall of 2012 seems surreal today. We experienced *so* much in a compressed period of time. A shocking diagnosis. Endless questions. Countless decisions. Paralyzing fear. Tremendous uncertainty. Overwhelming guilt. Debilitating fatigue. Gut-wrenching sorrow. Heartbreaking images. No plan. Sound familiar? Haven't we all experienced the same thing with our two-legged family members? So what is good for the goose is good for the gander, right? Prepare to care for your critters. Consider, in advance, how you will respond to a medical emergency or end-of-life care. Here are some elements of care:

- Pet insurance
- Financial planning
- Availability of caregivers

It's Time

After many months of watching Whisper decline, we had a tough decision to make. Our fifteen-year-old cat was struggling. Based on recent test results, her liver functions were marginal. We had just returned from the vet's office, unable to make the needed decision. For the past few weeks, JoAnne and I had both asked Whisper for a sign when she was ready to go. "Whisper, let us know when it's time." Thus far, no sign.

Once in the house, Whisper boldly walked into the kitchen. This caught our attention, because Whisper *never* went into the kitchen. But today, she was on a mission! She passed through the kitchen and finally stopped in the hallway. Once settled, she looked so peaceful. As we struggled to understand what was going on, we saw the sign. Whisper was sleeping under our chiming clock. It was time!

Inspiration

- Hospice and palliative care for critters
- Quality of life (yours and your critter's)
- Established limits of care
- Option of euthanasia
- Is it time?

Another consideration is this. Who will care for your critters if (when) you become ill or die? This is an extremely important question to ask and then answer. If you live alone, don't assume that your children, neighbors, or friends will figure it out. The transition of critter care should not become a crisis for your family and friends. Part of the responsibility of care is planning for the transition of care due to disability or death.

You can achieve a smooth transition of care in a variety of ways. Perhaps a friend or family member willingly offers to accept the responsibility for your critter. Some people choose to formalize the agreed transition in writing, perhaps even allocating money to cover anticipated expenses for the beloved critter. Or there are placement and matching services in some communities that assist with the transition upon the death of the guardian.

I recently heard of an innovative program sponsored by Colorado State University in Fort Collins, Colorado. Pets Forever is a nonprofit program for low-income seniors and disabled people who need assistance caring for their critters. Students in the service learning course provide the needed critter care. An added benefit of this course is the social connection between the student and the guardian of the critter. For more information, please check out the organization's website (csu-cvmbs.colostate.edu/vth/diagnostic-and-support/community-programs/pets-forever/Pages/default.aspx). This is an innovative model of care that will hopefully spread throughout the nation. The program cares not only for critters, but it cares for those of us who love critters as well. Fabulous!

To Summarize...

- The majority of households in the United States have at least one critter. Consequently, we must realize that, eventually, we will be caregivers to our critters. As with our other family members, proactive beats reactive every time!

- Critters are intuitive caregivers. As such, we have much to learn from our critter friends. Dogs, in particular, are artful in the practice of presence and nonverbal communication.

- Caregiving for critters and humans is remarkably similar. The physical, emotional, psychosocial, and spiritual impacts on caregivers are comparable. So do not underestimate the importance of preparing to care for your critter.

- Critters demonstrate an ability and willingness to receive care. This is an important lesson for all Boomers to learn. As we are confronted by chronic illness and increased longevity, we will require more care than we ever imagined. Learning to be a gracious care receiver will improve the process for all involved.

- If you have critters, you need to ensure the continuity of care if and when you become ill, disabled, or predecease your critter. If you are no longer able to care for your beloved critter, who will?

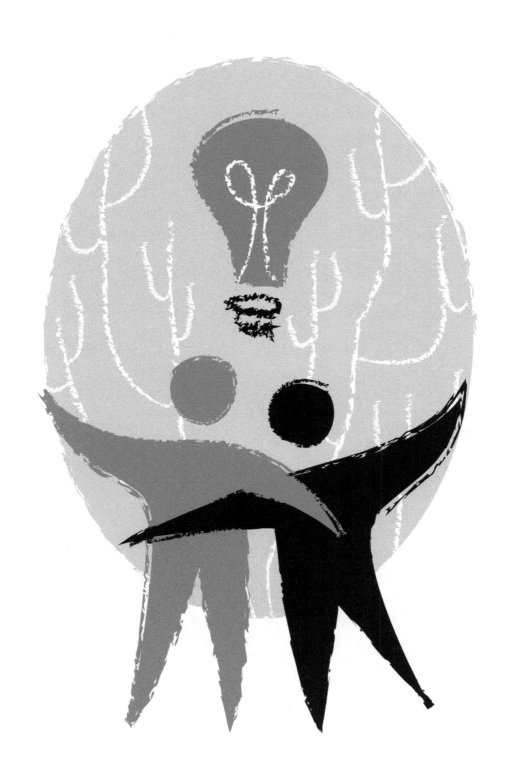

Assessment and Planning

An effective plan of care is rooted in reality. Whether a specific illness or advanced age, you must assess all aspects of the situation. Since you are not all knowing (sad but true), include all interested parties in the discussion. The changes prompted by advanced age and illness impact the entire family system. Create a forum in which all voices can be heard and all concerns addressed. Collaboration is the key to developing a successful plan of care. Now, before the left side of your brain hijacks the assessment and planning process, a word of caution. Assessing the situation is also an emotional process. Your approach to assessing the situation and subsequently developing a plan of care is critically important! If you fail to consider the feelings of your family members, you will live to regret the oversight. Instead, I'll explain the recipe for creating a collaborative, compassionate, and comprehensive plan of care. You will learn the needed ingredients to toss a SALAD! SALAD—good for you and your family!

Chapter 8

Assessment Process: Toss a SALAD!

In This Chapter...

- Now what?
- What are the ingredients for a healthy SALAD?
- What aspects of care do you need to assess?

Reality landed on your kitchen table this morning. Perhaps you received a call from your mother's neighbor. Your mother is not doing well. Or your doctor called with the pathology results. Positive. Regardless, your life just changed—*boom*! Now what? Remember our image of change (**Chapter 3**), the bridge? Today, you stand at the entry point of the bridge, staring into the vast unknown. You are paralyzed by fear. To move forward, you must acknowledge where you stand. Identify where you want to go. Create a plan to get there.

What do we *hope* for, and what do we *fear* when standing on the edge of the bridge? Well, if you're like the majority of folks in the United States, you *hope* to age in place (at home), and you *fear* the loss of independence. Illness and advanced age threaten to destroy your hope and confirm your fear. This dance between hope and fear must be understood to initiate an effective assessment and planning process. The logistical aspects of caregiving can then be discussed in a more compassionate way, realizing what the implications *mean* to the person.

We also need to recognize how caregivers and care receivers *feel* amidst all the changes and transitions generated by illness and advanced age. How we *feel* informs our behaviors and decisions related to aging and illness. Our understanding of the situation influences our preferred plan of care. It's not just about what we need; it's about what we *want* as well. A pragmatic approach produces a reasoned, logical plan of care. However, a pragmatic approach alone often fails to integrate the life-giving wants and desires of those involved. It fails to address the heart of the matter—*the people!* A better approach, a healthier approach, invites the consideration of wants, needs, hopes, and fears—a process that results in a healthy caregiving SALAD. We'll "toss" some ideas around on how this approach can help you and your family move through the assessment and planning process.

Caregiving Is a Continuous Process of Change

When, not if, someone in your family needs care, what will you do? What information do you need to create a comprehensive, compassionate, and effective plan of care? Preparing to care requires a comprehensive assessment of the current situation while acknowledging things will change in the future. Consequently, do not become enamored with your initial plan. It will change! You are standing on shifting sands. Caregiving is a continuous process of change resulting in disruptive transitions (**Chapter 3**). However, proactive beats reactive. Do your best to anticipate future needs.

Aging in Place

Where will you age? Where do you choose to age? Where do you want to be if (when) you become ill with a serious or progressive disease? If you are like most people in the United States, you will answer the above questions with a resounding, "I want to be *home*!" And rightly so. Home is where we belong. It is known. Home is our comfort zone filled with familiar people, stuff, and critters. Where else would I want to be? At home, I am in charge. In control. Independent.

This idea of staying and aging in your own home is called "aging in place." You've probably heard the term or read about it. Sounds like a good idea, right? Well, maybe. You see "aging in place" does not imply the quality of life enjoyed or endured as you age. It merely means that you are getting older where you stand. Could be good, could be bad. Please understand, this is *my* definition of the term "aging in place." There is a lack of consensus in the literature as to whether the term implies a positive quality of life or merely designates the location of aging. So I want to distinguish between "aging in place" and "aging *well* in place." To age *well* in place requires proactive assessment and planning. What served as a life-sustaining home at the age of forty may not serve you as well at eighty. Illness and advanced age are game changers. We must accommodate the changes by modifying the current environment or by transitioning to another place of residence.

Aging in Place (Jane's Definition!)

Aging in place means exactly that—you get older where you reside. Although most people claim they want to age in place, issues of safety may require a transition to another residence. Additionally, proximity to health care, community services, public transportation, and basic needs must be considered when evaluating the possibility of aging in place. To age *well* in place requires forethought and planning.

Definition

Aging in place is a concept that many organizations, businesses, and communities support. If we consider the concept from a societal perspective, aging in place contributes to the greater good. First, if people age in their place of choice, they're happier. People feel as if they're in control and independent. Second, aging in place makes financial sense. Typically, when a person transitions from home to a long-term care community, there is an increase in expenses. And, finally, as evidenced by the growth in home health services in the past ten years, serving the aging and the ill in their homes generates jobs in the community.

Despite the benefits of aging in place, personal and systemic, sometimes it's just not possible due to circumstances. This is particularly true for people who have not contemplated the possibility of illness or anticipated the reality of aging. If you want to age *well* in place, you *must* assess your situation and proactively plan for your ultimate demise.

Uninspired

Tripped Up by Stairs

When I worked in the petroleum business, transfers were the nature of the business. There was always significant mystery when moving. New people. New places. New commutes. And new neighbors. I was blessed when I moved to Houston. My next-door neighbors were lovely, welcoming people. They were my parents' age, and I enjoyed their spirit and presence in the neighborhood. I also marveled at their backyard. Gorgeous trees, flowers, and a water feature. This was their dream home. You could tell. They were there for the duration. Or so they thought.

Many years after moving to Houston, I noticed Tim putting a "For Sale" sign in the front yard. What? I couldn't believe my eyes. I ran out the front door and caught Tim before he walked into his garage. As I touched his shoulder, his eyes filled with tears. His heart was broken. And so was mine! I didn't want them to move. We sat down on the front steps, where he explained their situation.

Molly was diagnosed with Type 2 diabetes in her fifties. Now, twenty years later, she was suffering from neuropathy in her feet and hands. She could no longer walk up and down the stairs. It was just too painful. Since all of their bedrooms and full baths were on the second floor of their home, they decided to sell their home and move into a townhouse. Tim and Molly didn't want to move. They bought the house thinking it would be their last move. They wanted it to be their last move. At that, Tim laughed. The stairs weren't a concern when they bought the house twenty years before. Today, the stairs were the deal breaker.

To age well in place requires consideration of current and future needs. Don't be tripped up like Tim and Molly. Consider the "what ifs" and plan accordingly.

How you approach the assessment and planning process is often dependent on the *why* and the *who*. A crisis necessitates an immediate response. Sometimes a thoughtful assessment and plan will emerge after addressing the immediate needs. If you are hoping to avoid a future crisis, you must then take the time to carefully craft a plan of care. The *who* is fundamental to the assessment and plan of care. Beyond the current or future caregiving needs, you must consider the role of the *who* in the family and your relationship to the *who*. Are you concerned about your father, mother, spouse, or sibling? How will the person hear your concerns? Will the person have the same sense of urgency to create a plan of care? If you haven't thought about this, you should! You can easily offend, enrage, and alienate the person you want to help! Having been there and done that, I encourage you to be thoughtful in your approach.

Have a SALAD—It's Good for You!

To assist with the assessment and planning process, I have a suggestion for you. Have a SALAD! Wait. Don't rush off to the kitchen to chop veggies and lettuce. SALAD is a mnemonic for a process that assists in assessment and planning: Schedule, Ask, Listen, Assess, and Develop. Save the lettuce and croutons for later. We have other things to chew on right now.

To accurately assess a potential caregiving situation (or escalation of care), you need to invite all interested parties to the table for a chat. Be sure to include the person you are concerned about, the *who* in the equation. Care receivers need to have a voice in the plan of care, assuming they are able and willing. Your goal is to create a space for collaboration where all voices are welcome. All voices are heard. SALAD is a healthy way of assessing needs, wants, hopes, and fears. It is a recipe for creating a collaborative, compassionate, comprehensive plan of care. The recipe for a successful plan of care entails five essential "ingredients," or steps:

1. Schedule a meeting with all interested parties (care receiver, caregivers, and professionals).

2. Ask about the current situation. What's going on?

3. Listen to what is said and what is not (intuition).

Can We Start Over?

Our dad's stroke was a Red Flag Warning in many ways. Obviously, the stroke was shocking for all concerned. It also highlighted the fact that we were totally unprepared to care for our dad. No advance directives. No power of attorney. No medical durable power of attorney. Nothing! So we were determined to get all the paperwork in place to care for our dad. We had no other motivating factor other than our dad's well-being.

We consulted an attorney friend and determined the forms that needed to be filled out and signed. With papers in hand, we went to see our dad. We were on a mission! As it turned out, our dad was not as enthusiastic about the process as we were. He politely listened to our concerns. Glanced at the paperwork. And mumbled something about dealing with it later.

Over the next three years, my brother and I revisited the topic of paperwork (unsuccessfully) every time we went home to visit. The last time I broached the subject with my dad, he left little doubt that he was *not* signing the paperwork. We were sitting at the breakfast table, drinking coffee, and chatting. I decided to try one more time. I was about halfway through what I thought was an irresistible pitch when my dad rose from the table. He looked down at me and said in a very calm but firm voice, "I will *not* sign your papers today, tomorrow, or anytime in the future. Please do not bring up the subject again." Oh, and he emphasized his statement by slamming his fist on the breakfast table. A warm shower of coffee rained down as my coffee cup bounced off the table! I obviously needed to work on my delivery!

I tell this story not to vilify our dad. Rather, the story highlights the tremendous fear many people experience when illness or advanced age approaches. We fear losing control. Our dad knew we had his best intentions at heart. But he was not willing to relinquish any control. He was not ready to have his children making decisions for him. He was our dad. He was the patriarch of our family. And he was in control.

If I had the opportunity to speak to my dad today, I would ask if we could start over. Today, I would focus on alleviating his fears instead of getting his signature. Slowly but surely, I am getting older and a little wiser.

4. Assess abilities, disabilities, hopes, fears, needs, and wants to establish goals of care.

5. Develop, document, and execute a plan of care based on availability of needed resources.

To stay healthy, you need more than one SALAD. Sometimes, you have to "toss out" previous plans and develop new ones. As needs change, plans change. With each SALAD, you may be plus or minus some ingredients. Make the necessary adjustments to the recipe. Voila! Slightly different SALAD, but still life giving and life sustaining.

The SALAD process creates a collaborative community of care that honors the person being served as well as those who serve. Health care professionals provide needed information about the diagnosis and prognosis to make informed decisions regarding the logistical issues of care. The process allows for the sharing of hopes and fears, questions and concerns, needs and wants. Quite often, families are not on the same page. However, the initial gathering establishes a foundation of understanding and mutual respect. By sharing with, listening to, and honoring each other, families address more than the logistical issues of care. This approach reflects the sentiment that treating a condition or illness is not enough. We are called to serve persons—mind, body, and spirit. So I guess you could say that SALAD is heart healthy!

What to Ask

SALAD serves as the framework within which the actual assessment is done. Once you have gathered the interested parties, the inquiry begins in earnest. In step two, you determine what's going on. Pose the following questions to gather the information needed to generate the goals of care. The goals then drive the plan of care.

What Happened?

🔍 What is the cause for concern?

🔍 Is the need immediate or future?

🔍 Is there a consensus that a caregiving need/issue exists?

Who?

- Who is the potential care receiver?

- Does the care receiver live alone or with someone?

- What is the care receiver's role in the family (biological and functional)?

- What responsibilities need to be reassigned? Now? Future? Is the reassignment permanent or temporary? Who is willing and able to assume the responsibilities?

- Is the care receiver willing to receive help? If not, what are the sources of resistance? Personal, cultural, or family norm? Can the resistance be overcome?

- Will it be difficult to help the care receiver? Is the person belligerent? Rude? Offensive? Inappropriate?

What Care Is/Will Be Required?

- What is the nature of the disability or illness? Cognitive, physical, or mental?

- What are the diagnosis and prognosis?

- What level of care is required currently? Are professional caregivers needed in addition to family caregivers?

- Intensity of care? 24/7? Daily? Weekly?

- Which activities of daily living (ADLS) and instrumental activities of daily living (IADLs) does the care receiver need assistance with?

- Based on the prognosis, will the level of care escalate? If so, how quickly and to what level?

When and How Long?

- When is care needed? Immediately or in the future?

- How long will care be required?

ADLs and IADLs

ADLs are the basic, daily tasks that are used to determine the functional status of an individual. ADLS include bathing, dressing, toileting, transferring, continence, and feeding.

IADLs are not necessary for fundamental functioning, but they do allow persons to function independently. IADLS include shopping, housekeeping, meal preparation, accounting, transportation, and telephone.

Perspiration

Where?

- Where does the care receiver reside?

- What is the care receiver's proximity to friends and family?

- Where do the potential/current caregivers reside?

- Is the current residence a safe environment for the care receiver?

- Are property modifications required (ramps, grab rails, etc.)?

- Can the care receiver access services from the present location (health care, transportation, community services, basic needs)?

- What repairs, if any, does the current residence require to ensure a safe environment for the care receiver?

- Will future caregiving needs mandate a transition out of the home? If so, what options are available?

Are You Called to Care? Why?

- What is your relationship to the care receiver?

- What is your motivation to care? Love? Duty? By default? Responsibility? Family or cultural norm? Proximity to care receiver?

- What is the nature of your relationship with the care receiver? Loving? Conflicted? Contentious? Abusive? Volatile? Ambiguous?

- What are your limitations as a caregiver? Duration of care? Type of care? Location of care?

I have no doubt you will generate additional questions based on your specific situation. Every SALAD is unique based on the people involved and the compelling reason for care. Although I encourage the initial gathering of family and professionals, I realize this may not be possible. If you can't get everyone at the same table at the same time, utilize technology to gather the needed information from all interested parties. Phone calls, emails, Skype, videoconferences, etc. The goal is to invite and involve everyone critical to the creation of a compassionate, effective plan of care. Sometimes we have to be creative in how that happens! SALAD in not a rigid process. It is merely a guide to assist you in caring for a loved one. As any good cook will tell you, recipes are good to a point. Then you spice things up based on your personal preferences and taste.

After the Ask

Now that you have posed the important questions, gathered the needed information, and assessed abilities and disabilities, what next? Well, I'm glad you asked! According to our recipe, we are midway through step four. We now need to establish goals of care predicated on the hopes, fears, wants, and needs of the care receiver and the family. We are one step closer to developing a healthy plan of care. In **Chapter 9**, we'll discuss how the goals of care guide us through the frightening aftermath of change, bridge time.

To Summarize...

🔖 Most people desire to age in place. However, in order to age *well* in place requires forethought and planning. We can all age in place, but few do it well without a plan. You need not wait for a crisis before developing an effective plan of care. It is a given—you will require care as you age. Your family members will require care. So convene a gathering of interested parties. Discuss your hopes and fears. Your wants and needs. Your abilities and disabilities. If you want to age well, plan well.

🔖 Have a SALAD! It is a healthy approach to creating a collaborative, compassionate, comprehensive plan of care.

🔖 The assessment process addresses the who, what, when, where, why, and how of caregiving. It is also about recognizing the people behind the data. A plan of care is merely adequate if focused *strictly* on the logistical aspects of care. To develop a beneficial and honoring plan of care, you must know the person—mind, body, and spirit.

Chapter 9

Goals of Care: Products of a Healthy SALAD

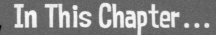

In This Chapter...

- What are goals of care?
- How do our foundational beliefs inform our goals of care?
- How does meaning transform our experience of suffering?
- What does it mean to witness the journey of illness and aging?

In **Chapter 8**, I introduced SALAD, a healthy approach to assess a caregiving situation and to develop a plan of care. The recipe for an effective plan of care includes the following essential ingredients or steps: schedule a meeting, ask for information, listen to responses, assess the information, and develop a comprehensive plan of care. In this chapter, it's time to generate goals of care based on the information you gathered through the assessment process. The goals of care will serve as guideposts to map the caregiving journey.

What are your goals of care? Well, it depends. Right? It depends on how you *see* the situation. It depends on your view of the world. It depends on your past experiences, your family legacy, and your cultural norms. Essentially, your goals of care emanate from your needs, wants, hopes, and fears. So your goals of care reflect these things:

- Your understanding of the diagnosis and prognosis. What should you anticipate as you walk across the transitional bridge (our image of change described in **Chapter 3**)?

- Your role in the caregiving scenario. Are you the person requiring care? Spouse or partner? Child? Doctor? Friend? What's your vested interest? What do you risk losing as the illness progresses or age continues to advance? Based on what you anticipate losing, are you hesitant to cross the bridge?

- Your understanding of illness and advanced age. Are you motivated to fight, to accept, or to despair? What do you envision on the other side of the bridge? Is the image hopeful or frightening? Compelling or repelling?

Realize the goals of care change as conditions change. Families must be willing and able to adjust the goals of care based on the current situation. Not what was. Rather, what is. When conditions change for the worse, this adjustment is obviously more difficult. Moving from one side of the bridge to the other requires a tremendous amount of courage. We are moving from the known to the unknown. We grieve the loss of what was and try to accept the reality of what is. Although the bridge serves as a path over the tumultuous waters of transition, it is not an easy journey. There will be moments of tremendous pain and suffering. That's when we need mile markers, the goals of care, to keep us on the straight and narrow. We also need a lure on the other side of the bridge to compel us to keep going, to push through the suffering and live beyond it. That compelling lure is *meaning*. Meaning transforms the potentially lethal experience of suffering. Meaning sustains us during times of trial and tribulation. Meaning motivates us to take the next step. To keep going. How do we find meaning in the midst of suffering? By faith. Faith provides the context within which to understand suffering and to struggle with the "whys" of life.

Goals of Care

Within health care, the primary goal of medicine evolved as medical technology evolved. Prior to 1900, patient comfort was the goal of care. With limited resources, cure was often not possible. Hence, the goal of care was to ensure the comfort and well-being of the patient. With the advent of medical technologies and medications in the twentieth century, the focus shifted from comfort to cure. Clinicians trained in the medical model of care focused on cure, sometimes at great expense (not just financially) to the patient and family. The curative measures were the source of suffering in many instances.

Since the 1970s, there has been a gradual shift in focus back to comfort as the goal of care prompted by the introduction of hospice care in the United States. Hospice recognizes that cure is not always possible. However, successful management of pain and symptoms is possible in most cases. The emphasis on alleviation of suffering enhanced the quality of life for the patient as well as the family. Slowly, very slowly, our health care systems and providers are realizing that it need not be *either* cure or comfort. It is both, cure *and* comfort. An illness can be aggressively treated with the hope for cure while effectively managing symptoms and pain. This integrated approach to health care is referred to as palliative care. *Palliative care* is the overarching philosophy of care that includes hospice care.

Both models of care focus on the prevention and alleviation of suffering, thus improving the quality of life for the patient and the family. Hospice and palliative care will be explored in detail in **Chapter 12**. In health care, as in families, goals of care evolve over time based on available resources, possibility of cure, values, and tolerance for and understanding of suffering.

Hospice and Palliative Care

Palliative care is an interdisciplinary approach to medical care focused on enhancing the quality of life for those challenged by advanced illness.

Hospice care is a type of palliative care reserved for those persons with terminal illness who are deemed to have less than six months to live.

Definition

Now is a good time to review our model of change and transition from **Chapter 3.** The metaphor of the bridge is helpful when discussing the goals of care. If you have a good memory, skip to the next paragraph. If you want a little refresher, continue on. The process of change and transition looks something like this. Imagine your life as a journey. The path is smooth and level, until something happens. *Change!* This change is represented by the entrance to a bridge. The bridge spans the space and time between what was (prior to change) and what will be (a new beginning). The transition, the aftermath of change, is the frightening time. *Bridge time.* The bridge transports you over the rough waters stirred up by the change in your life.

This is the time of uncertainty. The fog rolls in, clouding our perspective of life. Perhaps you've never been on this bridge before. Is it structurally sound? Are the boards strong or rotten? Can the bridge be trusted to carry you over the chasm of raging water? Good questions to ask. But don't hold your breath waiting for reassuring answers! To move on with your life often requires a leap of faith. Choosing to walk across the transitional bridge requires courage, determination, hope, and faith. So keep this image of change and transition in mind as we continue to talk about goals of care.

Within families, goals of care evolve with the changing condition of the patient (recovery or decline). Each change is followed by a time of transition, a period of adjustment. Needless to say, when dealing with a progressive illness, you have a lot of bridge time! In the case of advanced age or progressive illness, goals of care change as hope for cure or recovery wanes. As a family moves through the various stages of illness (diagnosis, acute, chronic, and terminal), the situation must be periodically reassessed to ensure viable goals of care. Granted, what is viable to you may not be viable to your parents. This is when families run aground. Illness and advanced age challenge the family system. However, the family does not always respond in unison, as a cohesive unit, because every person has a unique perspective. Consequently, goals of care can ignite heated debates within many families. These disputes arise because family members stand in different places on the transitional bridge. Each has a unique "view" of the situation. Each has a unique understanding. Each has valid points. Just knowing where people literally and figuratively stand serves to diffuse some potentially destructive arguments.

When to Revisit Goals of Care

- Change in health status of care receiver—for better or worse!

- Change in life expectancy—increased or decreased

- Change in care setting

- Change in decisional capacity of care receiver

- Change in treatment preferences

Perspiration

We often argue out of ignorance or the desire to be right. When it comes to goals of care, knowledge is power. Knowledge of the situation. Knowledge of the person being served. Knowledge of the disease process. Knowledge of the prognosis. Knowledge of your family. Additionally, it is not about being right or winning the point (tennis, anyone?). Keep in mind, we are talking about goals of *care*. Care being the operative word. How do you intend to care for your loved one, care for your family, and care for yourself? Enough said about your desire to be right? Good. Advantage, Jane!

What are your goals of care? Remember, goals of care will change as conditions change. But right now, what is important to you? What do you want? What do you need? What enables you to have an acceptable quality of life? From my personal as well as professional experiences, these are some common goals that might jump start your thought process:

- Curing the disease

- Relieving suffering

- Being surrounded by family and friends

- Being cared for at home

- Receiving effective pain and symptom management

- Continuing to work

- Living to see your first grandchild

- Enjoying a high quality of life

This list is far from comprehensive. However, it serves as a basis for discussion. Goals of care serve as guideposts throughout the caregiving journey. If you feel lost in the wilderness of medical technology and the myriad of treatment options, the goals of care help filter out what works for your family and what doesn't. For example, if your ultimate goal of care is cure, you will seek aggressive treatment options. If your primary goal is quality of life, you may not be willing to suffer the side effects of aggressive interventions. These are difficult questions that families across the country confront on a daily basis. The issues are mind numbing and heart wrenching. This is when solid goals of care can serve us well. In the example noted above, both perspectives regarding treatment options are valid, although diametrically opposed. The choices reflect the values of the individuals, the goals of care.

Your goals of care are the byproducts of who you are: your beliefs, your values, your lived experience, your role in the family, and your role in the caregiving experience. As a participant in the caregiving journey, you have a vested interest. You have something at stake. Something at risk. So goals of care also reflect your hopes and fears. This is true for all participants in the caregiving journey, family as well as professionals. Each person *sees* the journey uniquely through a "window on the world." By sharing our "views" with each other, we gain a panoramic perspective of the caregiving journey.

Pain and Suffering

We cannot discuss goals of care without specifically addressing the concern of pain and suffering. One of the greatest fears at the end of life is uncontrolled pain and suffering. Consequently, a primary goal of care is effective pain and symptom management. In order to achieve this very important goal, we must understand the concepts of pain and suffering. In common usage, the terms are used interchangeably. But suffering is quite different from pain. If I hit my thumb with a hammer, I will experience pain. My expectation is that the pain will subside in a matter of hours. In contrast, I suffer when something happens that doesn't make sense. I feel unjustly or undeservedly afflicted. Such as the diagnosis of a serious illness. Basically, my worldview is shattered. I am disoriented and unanchored. My experience of suffering is determined by how I *understand* the situation.

Example

Everyone Has an Opinion

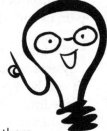

Walter was growing weary. He had been sitting on the couch for over an hour. He was ready to go back to bed. That last round of dialysis really threw him for a loop. Usually within a couple of hours, he was good to go. Not anymore. It was just getting harder and harder to put one foot in front of the other.

As he looked around the den, his heart went out to every person there. His wife. Daughter. Son. Grandson. And doctor. They met today to discuss the recent changes in his condition and figure out what to do. Well, Walter knew what he was going to do. But no one had asked him yet. Instead, his family was pushing the doctor for more ideas, more drugs, more options. Yep, there were other things that could be done, and everyone seemed to have an opinion, positive or negative, about each one. So far, there was no consensus about next steps.

His wife was adamant that Walter would stay at home. They had been married forty years, and she was going to care for him until his last breath. Bless her heart. Walter knew she was scared to live alone.

His daughter was determined to get another medical evaluation. This time, she wanted to take him across the country to a specialist she read about on the Internet. Yep, that's my girl. She can't imagine the world without her dad. So she keeps busy looking for options online.

His son had been guilted into coming to the meeting. He didn't have much to say, because in all honesty, he really didn't care. They had not spoken in over twenty years. It was nice he brought the grandson along. At least they had that little boy in common!

Then there was the doctor. Nice enough fellow, but he always got twitchy when Walter talked to him about stopping dialysis. You would have thought the doctor would have been able to talk about death. Yet he always avoided the subject. Instead, he offered new drugs, new diets, or the possibility of a kidney transplant. No surprise that the doctor and his daughter got along *really* well.

Walter might have considered some of these options a few years ago. Might have made some sense then. But not today. He was done. Done with this meeting. Done with dialysis. Done with life.

Everyone has an opinion. To be continued...

Pain and suffering are unique to each person. What I find mildly unpleasant, you might find excruciating. What causes me great suffering proves to be of no consequence to you. The point being, don't discount someone's claim of pain or suffering. Believe them!

Suffering is much more complex than physical pain, the typical focus of physicians. Suffering is described as an affliction of the "person," not just the body. A person suffers—the mind, body and spirit. Suffering emerges at the intersection of pain and belief. What does the pain mean? What do you think it means? There is also a futuristic element to suffering; a person's future is jeopardized, thus generating an overwhelming sense of futility. So, when suffering, a person has a sense the experience will never end. Therefore, suffering threatens to destroy the person.

Although the experience of suffering is unique to each person, there are characteristic aspects. Suffering challenges foundational beliefs and values, often to the point of disillusionment. The situation is literally beyond belief! There is often a sense of isolation, powerlessness, hopelessness, vulnerability, loss, and/or fear. It is when pushed to the extreme, when life seems senseless, that suffering threatens to destroy the person. Life is *meaningless*. There is no sense of purpose. If a person is suffering to this extreme, the goals of care will reflect that experience. The person just wants the suffering to end, often pleading with family and medical professionals to intervene. Later in the chapter, we will discuss the impact of suffering on the family, the witnesses to suffering. Suffering transforms the perspective of the care receiver and the caregivers. Often, it is the witnesses to suffering who plead to change the goals of care.

Walter's Situation

Let's revisit Walter and his family. Walter's worsening condition prompted the family meeting. As the family and doctor debated the various medical options, they missed the bigger issue. Walter is suffering. His journey has become meaningless over the past few years. Any changes in his goals of care are baseless if Walter is not seen and heard. Suffering need not be announced with thunder and lightning. Often, suffering is expressed as quiet despair, sitting on the couch.

Observation

Let's consider this idea of suffering using our image of the bridge. Where does suffering reside? Remember, I love a plan. If I know the specific location of suffering on my bridge, I can *plan* to avoid it! I'll step over that board and move on. Thank you very much! Nice idea, but suffering is not restricted to a particular part of the bridge. It can occur anywhere along the transitional bridge. This is why we feel so vulnerable and at risk throughout the caregiving journey. We're exposed to the elements with no place to hide! Not a pleasant part of the journey, to say the very least.

Extreme suffering, suffering beyond belief, heralds the dark nights of the soul. The moments in life when we can't find our way. Nothing is known. Fear is all consuming. All seems lost. There is no point of reference by which to navigate. We have lost our bearings, reluctant to move for fear of falling off the bridge. Are we doomed to perish on the bridge? Well, the good news is *no*! But whether you perish or persist is *your* choice. You must choose to seek the light, the glimmer of hope on the far side of the bridge that serves to guide your next steps. You may forever remain perplexed by your experience on the bridge, questioning *why* you had to suffer. However, by focusing on the guiding light in your life (that which gives you a greater meaning and purpose), you are able to move through moments of suffering to live beyond them. Yes, you will suffer. But you will not be destroyed. Meaning, in the greater context of life, penetrates and illuminates our darkest nights.

> *To live is to suffer; to survive is to find some meaning in the suffering.*
>
> Friedrich Nietzsche, nineteenth-century German philosopher
>
> Quote

What Guides, Grounds, and Sustains You?

Fine. So, how do we change our experience of suffering from one of potential annihilation (meaningless suffering) to one of positive transformation (moving across the bridge)? Where do we go for answers? We go to that which historically sustains us during the times that try our souls. We rely on our foundational beliefs to help us make sense of our circumstances: faith, religion, spirituality, beliefs, values, morals, ethics, and/or worldview. Whatever you call it, it is the guiding and sustaining set of beliefs that serve as your litmus test for life. This is the solid ground on which you stand when the earth shakes and the walls come tumbling down. It is the point of reference, the guiding light that we seek when standing on the bridge.

At this point in our discussion, I know my dad is frowning somewhere. You see, my dad thought it inappropriate to discuss sex, politics, money, or religion outside of the family. One of our family norms. Oh well, one of the many family norms I have modified over the years! If, by chance, you are hesitant to discuss religion and spirituality with a stranger, let me assuage your fears. Whatever you believe to be true, I honor and respect. My intent is not to convince, coerce, or convert you. Instead, I merely invite you to consider how your faith serves you during times of change, transition, and suffering.

Let's first define spirituality and religion. Oh, that should be easy! Spirituality and religion are terms and concepts that defy concise definition. There is no "one" definition for either term that is acceptable to all. Historically, the traditional distinction was that spirituality referred to personal faith, and religion was associated with institutionalized faith. So spirituality was more psychological and religion was more sociological. In short, both terms are ambiguous and must be defined by the person using the terms. You may describe yourself as spiritual but not religious. Or you may choose to describe yourself as religious. Again, your choice. I honor both descriptors. I prefer not to debate the labels. Instead, I long to know the *person*. So, for the purposes of brevity and inclusion, I will refer to *all* guiding, grounding, and sustaining belief systems as "faith." All are welcome and wanted in the conversation.

We now need to consider the functional nature of faith. What purpose does faith serve? Faith is concerned with how we come to terms with the ultimate issues of life, such as death, suffering, tragedy, evil, and pain. What does it mean? When we lack clarity and certainty, faith often guides, grounds, and sustains as we seek to understand. I am not suggesting that we use our faith to justify suffering. Instead, faith provides a context in which to understand the experience of suffering. Faith helps us place suffering in the broader context of the entirety of our existence. The meaning is not so much about the momentary experience of suffering but the meaning of life (remember

It's Not About You

Several years ago, I presented a program on spirituality and health to a class of nursing students. As always, I enjoyed the experience. As I packed up to leave at the end of the day, a young woman approached asking if I had time to chat.

The student remarked that I had done an "adequate" job of discussing spirituality in health care. Based on her facial expression and body language, I could tell she was primed for a fight! I had stepped on her spiritual toes somewhere along the way. So I asked if she had any concerns about the program. This led to a very interesting discussion.

She was very offended that I had excluded her from the conversation. Unbeknownst to me, she was an atheist. The topic of spirituality was of no interest or consequence to her. She advised that I be a bit more sensitive the next time I presented the subject. She then folded her arms and sat back. Waiting for a response.

I expressed my regret that she missed the initial invitation for *all* to join in the discussion. Regardless of a person's faith tradition or belief system, I invited everyone to join the conversation. Whatever guides, grounds, and sustains a person—that was a system of belief for the purposes of that day's discussion. I acknowledged that my definition of spirituality was much broader than others. My class; my rules.

However, debating definitions was not my thing. I was more concerned about her self-absorption. I reminded her that as a nurse (assuming she graduated), she would be serving a diverse population. Different ethnicities, races, nationalities, ages, genders, *and* spiritual beliefs. As a nurse, it mattered not what she believed to be true. What mattered is what her patient believed to be true. To serve well, she didn't have to agree with the perspective of her patient. But she did have to honor the perspective of the person. So the nursing student had missed the essential point of the presentation. It wasn't all about her!

I said this in what I thought was a caring and compassionate way. But I also stressed the importance of seeking first to understand, then to be understood. Slowly, a smile spread across the nurse-to-be's face, and she nodded. Her "aha moment" arrived. With an open mind and open heart, we enjoyed an incredible conversation over the next two hours.

It's amazing what happens when you don't have an agenda. Remember, your mission is *not* to convince, coerce, or convert. Instead, we are called to listen, understand, and serve.

A Ray of Hope

Walter decided enough was enough. His family could continue the conversation with the doctor. No one seemed to care about what he thought at this point anyway. Oh well. They would know soon enough that he had no intention of continuing this agonizing process.

As Walter was preparing to stand and leave the room, his grandson walked over and sat beside him on the couch. Walter was surprised by how much he had grown in the past year. At seven years of age, his grandson was pretty tall! Even more surprising, Walter saw a bit of himself in the boy! Although Walter and his own son never clicked, there was something about his grandson that grabbed his heart. Something special. So there was no way Walter could refuse his grandson's invitation to his birthday party in two weeks.

Two weeks. Walter knew he could hang on for two weeks. This was important to his grandson. And it was important to Walter. Something to look forward to.

Example

the scene previously described on the bridge). Faith then seems to be a compelling way to cope as it allows for the reframing of the situation and possible discernment of meaning in the midst of suffering. Faith "works" because it gives people a sense of meaning and control.

This sounds lovely. Faith supports and sustains us during the tough times. Faith is our window on the world that provides clarity, focus, and meaning in the midst of suffering. Our understanding of the situation within the larger context of life disarms suffering, thus mitigating the potential threat of destruction. Lovely, indeed, until your search for meaning proves futile. You stand on the bridge, peering into the darkness. No light to be seen. What then?

There are times in life, tragic situations, when our depth of suffering defies explanation. This type of suffering tests fundamental beliefs, often shattering our window on the world and necessitating the reconstruction of faith at some point. Such times of self-examination and subsequent transformation, although difficult, can ultimately result in a stronger faith. It is not how most of us would choose to become more faithful. However, intense suffering often spawns tremendous personal growth and transformation.

Finally, we must acknowledge that faith can also be a punitive and thus detrimental force in the midst of change, transition, and suffering. If you believe your suffering to be deserved, your goals of care will reflect that understanding as well. Flip back to **Chapter 4**, the story of the young woman who believed cervical cancer was punishment for her sin of adultery. Therefore, she did not seek treatment. I have no intention of condoning or condemning her faith. However, we need to seriously consider the consequences of her faith, the meaning given to her illness. Is there a way to respectfully invite her to understand the diagnosis of cancer in a different way? Could her experience of cancer actually serve to deepen her faith by expanding her view of life? I don't know. But I do believe it's worthy of consideration.

The Role of Witness

As caregivers, personal or professional, we participate in the journey of caregiving. We experience the highs and lows, the ups and downs, and sometimes the sideways! But our journey is quite different from that of the care receiver. It is not *our* journey. Rather, we serve as witnesses and companions—an incredibly important role indeed. To witness the suffering of others requires commitment, compassion, and courage.

The role of witness is significantly impacted by the goals of care. The goals of care often determine *what* we witness. For example, consider the diagnosis of ovarian cancer. If the goal of care is cure, then we will witness aggressive treatments with possible side effects. If the goal of care is comfort, we will witness the advance of terminal cancer and ultimately death. In either case, we will witness pain, suffering, change, and significant loss. The disease is not ours. The pain is not ours. But we are vicariously affected as we witness the suffering of another person.

As witnesses, we must realize what is within our control and what is not. If you serve as a caregiver, you obviously have a caring and compassionate heart. So when you witness your care receiver hurting or suffering, you want to *fix it*, right? Well, with advancing age, or chronic or terminal illness, you can't fix it! Instead, you will witness the consequences of the condition. For me, this is *the* hardest aspect of companioning our loved ones and being witness to the journey. It requires a tremendous amount of courage to be present to the pain and suffering of another being (human or critter)

Coming of Age

Walter was true to his word. He attended his grandson's birthday party. It had been a rough couple of weeks, but Walter was determined to be there. The scene was bittersweet. Watching his grandson, he saw the promise and hope of youth. Such a stark contrast to Walter's situation of little promise and very little hope. Feeling a bit melancholy, Walter decided to go outside and sit on the porch. He wouldn't be missed.

Imagine Walter's surprise when his grandson sat down beside him on the porch swing. His grandson didn't say anything. Instead, he slipped his small hand into Walter's, and they sat. Swinging gently on a summer afternoon. No words were exchanged. But through the connection of hands and hearts, the emotions flowed. As the tears streamed down Walter's cheeks, his grandson came of age. To witness the suffering of a loved one requires incredible courage. Walter's grandson was courageous that day.

Pure Genius!

knowing there is nothing to be done to change the course of the disease. However, it is also a sacred honor, a calling, to companion those we love to the end of the road. To be present.

Remember the story of Job in the Hebrew Bible? This is the timeless story of inexplicable loss and undeserved suffering. The story of every man and every woman. My favorite part of the story deals with Job's friends. Do you recall how Job's three friends showed up to sit with him? Job was sitting on an ash heap, scraping his wounds with shards of pottery. For seven days, Job reflected on his fate. His friends never said a word. Not a word! What an incredible gift offered by Job's friends. For seven days, his friends resisted the temptation to try to "fix" Job. They made no suggestions. Asked no questions. And offered no justifications of his fate. For seven days, they were stellar witnesses. *Then* they began to speak. That's when things started going south, as is so often the case. But, in their defense, it's hard to witness the suffering of a friend.

Witnessing takes a toll. Particularly in cases of refractory pain (resistant to drugs or treatments) and existential suffering (struggling with the reality of mortality), witnesses suffer to the extreme as well. This often causes the family and health care providers to revisit the goals of care. For example, a previous goal of mental acuity may be supplanted by the goal of adequate pain management (higher doses of pain medications). Suffice it to say, the goals of care evolve as the journey unfolds. The care receiver, caregivers, and health care professionals must work collaboratively to generate appropriate, beneficial, and compassionate goals of care.

To Summarize...

- Goals of care reflect the needs, wants, hopes, and fears of the care receiver and the family. The goals serve as guideposts as conditions change and the caregiving journey unfolds. Goals evolve as the needs and desires change.

- One of the greatest fears at the end of life is uncontrolled pain and suffering. Consequently, a primary goal of care is effective pain and symptom management. In order to achieve this goal, we must understand the distinction between pain and suffering. Additionally, we need to recognize the relationship between suffering and meaning. As Friedrich Nietzsche said, "To live is to suffer; to survive is to find some meaning in the suffering."

- Meaning in the midst of suffering is derived from our foundational beliefs, our faith. These guiding and sustaining principles do not justify the pain and the suffering experienced. Instead, our faith provides a larger context within which to understand the suffering. Our faith is the guiding light that illuminates the path across the transitional bridge.

- As caregivers, we are witnesses to pain and suffering. As such, we are deeply affected by the journey. It is important to understand that the goals of care affect all involved. Consequently, the care receiver, caregivers, and medical professionals must work collaboratively to develop, and modify as needed, effective goals of care.

Chapter 10

Develop, Document, and Execute a Plan of Care: Dress the SALAD

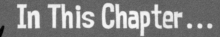

In This Chapter...

- What community resources are needed, available, and/or preferred to achieve the goals of care?

- What personal resources are needed, available, and/or preferred to achieve the goals of care?

- What professional resources are needed, available, and/or preferred to achieve the goals of care?

- What financial resources are needed, available, and/or preferred to achieve the goals of care?

It is now time for the final step in the SALAD process. We are well on our way to creating a healthy plan of care! We assessed the situation in **Chapter 8**. We established the goals of care in **Chapter 9**. So we now have all the necessary ingredients to complete our SALAD. The remaining task in the recipe is to "dress the SALAD," using available, needed, and/or preferred resources.

The goals of care drive the plan of care, obviously. However, availability of needed or preferred resources is often the determining factor in the plan of care. The goals of care may initially seem reasonable but ultimately prove impossible due to circumstances. As conditions change, we will encounter similar "reality checks" along the way. Remember, this is not a one-time process. With every change prompted by aging and/or illness, we have to reassess, revise goals of care, and tweak the plan of care. It is an iterative process.

If we are to age well, we must plan well. For some, this means relinquishing or revising dreams due to physical, cognitive, or financial changes. I hope the story of Henry and Carmen will motivate you to plan well. You may be living the dream today. But as you age, your dream can become a nightmare of unimagined challenges and obstacles. Proactive beats reactive every time!

SALAD Process

1. Schedule a meeting with all interested parties (care receiver, caregivers, and professionals).

2. Ask about the current situation. What's going on?

3. Listen to what is said and what is not (intuition).

4. Assess abilities, disabilities, hopes, fears, needs, and wants to establish goals of care.

5. Develop, document, and execute a plan of care based on availability of needed resources.

IMPORTANT!

Meet Henry and Carmen

Several years ago, I spent a week on the northern California coast. I quickly fell in love with the people, the place, and the pace of life. I was grateful for the slower pace, as it allowed the time needed to appreciate the moment. Savor the sights. And meet amazing people.

I opted to stay for a week in a tiny little village right on the coast. I learned from the locals that nine hundred people lived there year-round. Based on the season, the village would expand or contract. In a week's time, I managed to meet a significant number of locals as I frequented the restaurants, shops, farmers market, and various parks. The second day of my visit, I stopped by the Visitor's Information Center to pick up trail maps and to get the scoop on local fare and activities. As it turned out, I gathered more than information about the village. I gained a profound respect for the timeless real estate mantra, "location, location, location."

Henry was working the desk at the Visitor's Information Center the day I stopped by. He appeared to be in his late seventies. Since I was in no hurry (I had embraced the local pace by then), I asked Henry what brought him to the village. I wanted to know his story. There was no one else in the office, so we had time to chat. And Henry needed to chat. He needed someone to listen to his story. He needed to grieve and to mourn the loss of a dream.

Henry was a retired pastor. For forty years, he served congregations in the Sacramento area. He and his beloved wife of over fifty years raised three children who were now scattered across the country. Occasionally, the children returned to California for a much-welcomed visit. However, Henry realized his children were busy working, raising their own children, and living life. It would be nice to see them more often, but Henry and Carmen didn't press the issue. Their children had limited time and money right now. Since retirement, it was easier for Henry and Carmen to hop a plane for a visit. At least it had been. Things had changed recently.

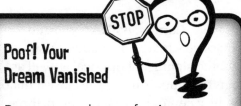

Poof! Your Dream Vanished

Be sure your dream of retirement is rooted in reality. Your dream can vanish in a heartbeat if you fail to anticipate future health care needs. You must plan well to live the dream. Be proactive and realistic.

WATCH OUT!

Five years ago, Henry and his wife, Carmen, decided it was time to leave congregational ministry and enjoy the fruits of their labors. Every summer of their married life, they had spent two weeks on the California coast. So, not surprisingly, they dreamed of moving to one of their favorite spots. They knew exactly where they wanted to live. Not just the village, but the exact house! For years, they monitored the real estate listings hoping the house would go on the market. As luck would have it, the house went up for sale just about the time Henry had the urge to retire. Thinking that was a sign of some sort, Henry and Carmen made the big decision to retire and move to the coast. They were ready to live their dream!

As Henry shared his story, his body language and intonation did not reflect a man living his dream. Henry looked weary and incredibly sad. There were several times during the conveyance of his story that his eyes filled with tears.

Although we had just met, I couldn't leave without inquiring about his apparent anguish. I felt he needed and wanted to talk. And I was willing and able to listen.

Community Resources

I thanked Henry for sharing his story. I don't meet many people who claim to be living their dream. Yet I sensed an intense sadness as he spoke. Was there something going on that he wanted to talk about it? At this invitation, Henry took a deep breath. Nodded his head in the affirmative. Then I heard the rest of the story.

Last year, Carmen had experienced a massive stroke. Consequently, she suffered significant physical as well as cognitive impairment. The closest major medical center is in Sacramento, three hours away by car. If they had lived in Sacramento when the stroke happened, Carmen would have received the needed care in short order, possibly minimizing the resultant brain damage. Henry felt so guilty! They never thought about the "what ifs" of a medical emergency. Before Carmen's stroke, they both enjoyed excellent health. They should have known better. They should have planned better! *If* they hadn't moved, Carmen would still be enjoying life. As it was, she struggled to get through the day. And so did Henry.

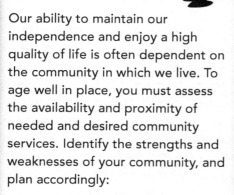

Community Resources

Our ability to maintain our independence and enjoy a high quality of life is often dependent on the community in which we live. To age well in place, you must assess the availability and proximity of needed and desired community services. Identify the strengths and weaknesses of your community, and plan accordingly:

- Medical services (hospitals, clinics, home and community-based services [also known as HCBSs], etc.)
- Public transportation
- Senior centers—programs, locations, services
- Adult day care centers
- Area agency on aging
- Senior nutrition programs (Meals on Wheels)

Inspiration

Personal Resources

Currently, the village did not serve Henry and Carmen well from the standpoint of available community services. I wondered how Henry managed to care for his wife. With Carmen's cognitive and physical impairment, Henry had his hands full. Since their children lived outside of California, they were not available on a daily basis to help Henry. I was concerned that Henry was trying to do everything by himself. The role of primary caregiver could easily compromise his health as well.

I asked Henry if he had a supportive group of friends to help out from time to time. Henry shared that they were blessed with very dear friends in the village, people they had met over the past forty years when vacationing on the coast. Many wanted to help, but they had their own health issues. In fact, the core population of the village consisted of retirees over the age of 60. The children in the village typically moved to the city after graduation from high school seeking employment and excitement. The folks in between the children and the retirees were business owners in the village who were trying to make a living. Consequently, Henry had few people he could rely on. He was incredibly thankful for his volunteer work at the Visitor's Information Center. Every Wednesday, Carmen's best friend stayed with her *all* day, giving Henry a much-needed break. Wednesdays were his saving grace. He was thankful that Carmen's friend finally convinced him the break would be good for both Carmen and Henry. Even so, Henry felt guilty when he was away from her.

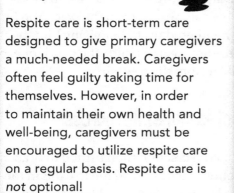

Respite Care— *Not* Optional

Respite care is short-term care designed to give primary caregivers a much-needed break. Caregivers often feel guilty taking time for themselves. However, in order to maintain their own health and well-being, caregivers must be encouraged to utilize respite care on a regular basis. Respite care is *not* optional!

Observation

Listening to Henry, I desperately wanted to help him! This is *not* what Henry and Carmen had planned. Since I don't hide my emotions very well, Henry saw the concern in my eyes and quickly apologized for "dumping" his worries on me. He and Carmen were figuring things out, one step at a time. Although he was having a tough day, Henry thought they were handling the situation pretty well overall.

Even though help was limited, Henry never felt alone. He relied on his faith for support and sustenance. That was one thing he could access anytime, anywhere, and any day. Immediately following the stroke, he had been incredibly angry. Literally screaming "Why?" to the heavens and feeling abandoned by his god. Gradually, he discovered the courage to face the reality of the situation. Carmen had a stroke. Life would never be the same. Their dream evaporated in a heartbeat. Thus, he had a choice to make. Rage or respond. He was proud to say that he chose to respond—to bounce back and meet the challenges of life head on. The journey was far from smooth. But they were taking it one step at a time and trusting the process. He recalled giving similar advice to those in his congregations in the past. And he remembered his father giving him the same advice as a child. The acorn doesn't fall far from the tree, eh?

Professional Resources

Our conversation then turned to practical matters. Henry asked me to explain the mysteries of Medicare. I laughed out loud! I am well versed in many aspects of aging and illness. However, Medicare remains a mystery. When in doubt, I rely on esteemed colleagues who specialize in Medicare. But I was curious about Henry's experience of Medicare.

Personal Resources

What personal resources serve you well when life happens? Who is there for you? What life experiences inform your responses? What foundational beliefs sustain you during times of trial? How do you choose to respond to life?

 Family

 Friends

 Neighbors

 Colleagues

 Faith community

 Community members

 Attitude

 Spirituality/religion

 Resilience

Previous life experiences

Family legacies

Inspiration

After Carmen's stroke, Henry spent hours on the phone with Medicare trying to understand the available services and benefits. Recently, he realized Medicare had not a *clue* what it meant to live in a village, isolated from medical centers and supportive health care services. The last three times he called Medicare, the representative encouraged Henry to take advantage of the in-home services covered by Medicare. Each time, Henry listened patiently as the representative sang the praises of home and community-based services, service providers that provide care in the home. Each time, Henry asked the representative if they were familiar with the California coast. And each time, Henry had to explain that no matter how much Medicare would pay, there were *no* service providers within 150 miles of their home. There was *no one* to pay! A stunned silence ensued, followed by a muttered apology and best wishes.

Henry was very familiar with the variety of senior services and health care options in Sacramento. He companioned aging and ill members of his church for forty years. Henry did a good job of referring his members to beneficial experts and organizations. Families dealing with dementia were directed to the Alzheimer's Association. Seniors, or adult children of seniors, concerned about finances and legal issues were encouraged to seek wise counsel from financial planners and elder law attorneys. There were even companies in Sacramento that helped families "get organized" as individuals transitioned from houses into long-term care communities. Many of his members cared for aging parents in other states. In those cases, geriatric care managers served as the eyes, ears, hands, and feet on the ground for the long-distance caregivers. And certainly Henry counseled many individuals and families about the blessings of hospice and palliative care. So Henry knew exactly what he and Carmen needed and wanted. He also knew those services were not available in the village.

Housing Resources

Henry decided we needed a cup of coffee and more comfortable seating. With coffee in hand, we moved to the rocking chairs outside on the porch. The fresh air, caffeine, and change of scenery recharged the conversation. It was then that Henry shared the source of the sadness I sensed initially. In the past week, he and Carmen finally admitted what their children had been telling them for the past year. They needed to move. Their dream home in the

Professional Resources

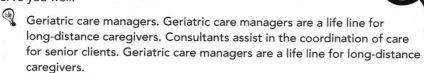

Illness and aging pose specific challenges. Hence, we need professionals who specialize in the specifics of illness and aging. Depending on your situation, the following professionals can serve you well:

- **Geriatric care managers.** Geriatric care managers are a life line for long-distance caregivers. Consultants assist in the coordination of care for senior clients. Geriatric care managers are a life line for long-distance caregivers.

- **Disease-specific agencies.** Agencies provide educational information related to the disease process. Many agencies offer support groups, educational programs, hotlines, counseling services, and referral information.

- **Medical professionals.** As we age, we will become all too familiar with a variety of medical specialists and health care providers. Our options for care ultimately depend on where we live, our insurance coverage, and our financial resources.

- **Home and community-based services (HCBSs).** Service providers come to the home, allowing clients to remain independent as long as possible. Services can be either medical or nonmedical in nature.

- **Hospice and palliative care.** Discussed in detail in **Chapter 11.**

- **Pastoral care professionals.** Clergy, chaplains, spiritual directors, and lay ministers address the spiritual needs of care receivers and family members.

- **Eldercare financial planners.** As we age, we have different financial goals and needs. Financial planners who specialize in eldercare issues focus on the specific needs of the aging population.

- **Elder law attorneys.** Specialized legal advice is beneficial when contemplating financial wills and medical directives.

- **Patient navigators.** Families that are befuddled and bemused by the complexities of the health care system benefit greatly by these knowledgeable guides.

- **Placement specialists.** When considering the myriad of available housing options, you are wise to consult with an expert who is knowledgeable about the site, the staff, and the management of each location.

- **Moving specialists.** Organizational specialists can help clients downsize, conduct estate sales, and relocate.

village was multilevel with all the full baths on the second level. After a year of rehab and physical therapy, Carmen still had great difficulty navigating the stairs. Certainly a cause for concern. The last thing they needed was for Carmen to fall on the stairs. Additionally, Carmen needed access to medical and therapeutic services on a regular basis. The drives to and from Sacramento were exhausting for both Henry and Carmen. The day-to-day routine of care was taking a toll on Henry. It was time to admit that he needed help caring for Carmen. They had to move. So, one decision down. One remained. Where? Where should they move?

At this point, Henry excused himself to assist another person interested in the village life. While he was away, my thoughts drifted to Carmen. Bless her heart! I wondered how she felt about all the events of the past year. Like Henry, the stroke changed her life forever. Unexpected. Unwanted. Unwelcome. Their dream of living on the coast had turned into a nightmare. Did she feel guilty? Angry? Frustrated? Betrayed? Depressed? Sad? I was sure she felt all that and so much more.

My thoughts of Carmen were interrupted by Henry's return. We picked up where we left off. Where to move. Their daughter insisted that Henry and Carmen move in with her. She had plenty of room and would welcome her parents with open arms. It all sounded lovely, but Henry and Carmen didn't want to be a burden. Plus, their daughter lived in New Jersey. They didn't know another soul in New Jersey! So that option was nixed quickly. The obvious choice (in Henry's opinion) was Sacramento. They had lots of friends in the city. Based on their experience of the past year, a supportive community of friends was not just wanted but was needed for the duration. They also knew Sacramento inside and out. They could easily slide back into the community and quickly feel "at home." Although it wasn't their "dream" retirement, there was a comforting sense of "the known" in Sacramento.

Consequently, Henry was busy exploring the various housing options in Sacramento. He and Carmen wanted to live close to Carmen's doctors and therapists. But, even more importantly, they wanted to be close to friends and their faith community. They outlined their preferred part of town and then met with a placement specialist. Henry and Carmen had never explored the various long-term care communities in Sacramento, thinking they would retire on the coast. But, the new reality mandated a new plan. This time, they wanted a plan that would accommodate current and future changes in their physical and cognitive abilities. They needed to consider the "what ifs" and plan accordingly. Older and wiser indeed!

Financial Resources

The morning passed by quickly with Henry. I felt as if I had known him forever by the time we parted ways. Before I left to continue my journey, Henry felt compelled to pass along some fatherly advice. He realized, based on my gray hair and hard-earned wrinkles, the question of retirement was or would be of concern. He cautioned me to be realistic about retirement. To consider the "what ifs" carefully. To select a community in which aging is supported and served. He wanted to save me the heartache that he and Carmen were experiencing—the heartache of relinquishing a lifelong dream in exchange for the harsh reality of advanced age, illness, and disability.

His final words of wisdom concerned the hefty price tag of aging and illness. As with all aspects of aging, knowledge is power. This is particularly true when it comes to financing retirement and the aging process. If we fail to adequately save and invest for retirement and the increased levels of physical and cognitive care, our options are severely limited. We can reduce our financial risk by purchasing a variety of insurance policies: life insurance, long-term care insurance, and health insurance. However, one size doesn't fit all. We must explore the options to determine the advisability of each.

Being of my parents' generation (Traditionalists), Henry was all about saving and investing for the future. The Great Depression left a major impression on those who struggled to survive. Thoughtful consideration accompanied every purchase. Frugality was the societal norm. Although Henry and Carmen had been financially conservative throughout their marriage, Henry was concerned (and rightly so) about the increased expense of a long-term care community. The key to their financial security resided in their ability to sell their home on the coast prior to moving to Sacramento. However, houses in the village were not moving. Henry couldn't afford a mortgage payment plus the fees associated with an assisted living community. At this point, he just hoped to hang on until a buyer showed up.

Housing Resources

What are the options for housing as we age?

- Aging in place. You get old where you stand. To age *well* in place requires planning.

- Living with family. Many people opt to move in with a family member when aging or illness precludes living alone. Sometimes this is the only financially viable option. Be prepared for some interesting family dynamics.

- Granny pods. Modular units that serve to house one person typically. Zoning restrictions, HOA covenants, and available space are often limiting factors for this option.

- Long-term care communities (independent living, continuing care retirement communities, assisted living, skilled nursing, and memory care). The best option depends on the level of care required, anticipated levels of care, and financial ability to pay for the services.

- Affordable housing options (subsidized rental options). Low-income housing offers affordable housing options. Availability varies depending on your location.

- Cohousing community. A cohousing community is an intentional community designed to share resources, share expenses, and share the experiences of life. This concept is becoming very popular nationally.

- Personal emergency response systems. These systems enable previously "at risk" individuals to remain independent. Truly a comfort for long-distance caregivers to know their loved one is being monitored for falls or medical emergencies.

- Adaptive devices (assists those with vision, hearing, and physical impairments). Technological and adaptive devices allow those with disabilities to remain independent and autonomous.

Eventually, Henry needed to get back to his post in the Visitor's Information Center, and I needed to be on my way. We shared the hug of good friends— both arms wrapped tightly around each other. Henry thanked me and said he felt considerably better after unloading. I thanked Henry for trusting me enough to dump! Laughing, we parted ways. As I strolled through the village, I reflected on my conversation with Henry. I realized my gift to Henry was my presence and willingness to listen. I wondered if Henry realized the gift he bestowed on me—his poignant, raw, *real* story. Priceless! Henry's words of wisdom increase the likelihood that I will live my dream. I share this story with you in the hope that Henry will inspire you as well. Then we can all thank Henry when we are living the dream!

The Lessons of Henry and Carmen

In the introduction of this book, I highlighted the importance of proactive planning. If we are to age well, we *must* prepare to care for ourselves and for our families. Just in case you missed it, the theme of proactive planning is mentioned in every chapter of this book. SALAD serves as the recipe for successful planning, itemizing the ingredients and the steps required to create a healthy plan of care. How I wished Henry and Carmen had "tossed" a SALAD *before* moving to the coast of California. Lack of realistic assessment and planning resulted in limited options when the unexpected health care crisis happened. Henry and Carmen had no wiggle room. The needs were immediate and extensive. The urgency was high. And resources were limited. This was the perfect storm for Henry and Carmen. Perfectly horrible! Without a viable plan, Henry was knee-deep in alligators and the tide was rising! Henry and Carmen had a dream, but they failed to develop a viable plan of care.

Henry's story highlights the importance of identifying the needed, available, and preferred resources required to achieve the goals of care. It matters not what we need and want if the services are not available. So we are wise to anticipate the possible physical and cognitive challenges associated with advanced age or illness and to plan appropriately. Henry and Carmen did not anticipate the possibility of a life-changing medical condition. Instead, they were mesmerized by their dream of retiring on the coast. And who wouldn't be? It's a lovely dream! But we have to remember that to age *well* requires thoughtful, proactive planning. We can't anticipate everything

Financial Resources

A daunting challenge for Boomers is funding our retirement and aging process. An honest evaluation of your current and future financial resources is mandatory to develop a viable plan of care. What resources do you have to cover the medical expenses and associated costs of aging? What community, state, and federal resources exist to assist the aging population?

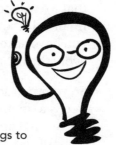

- Personal savings and investments. Do you have adequate savings to fund your retirement? If not, what do you plan to do?

- Retirement plans and pensions. Does your current employer provide retirement and pension plans? Are you taking advantage of the investment and savings options?

- Financial planners. Have you consulted with a financial planner to ensure you have accurately assessed your future financial needs?

- Long-term care insurance. Many financial planners believe a financial plan is incomplete without LTC insurance. Just know, this type of insurance is becoming very expensive. If interested, check it out sooner rather than later!

- Medicare. Check out the Medicare website for information about the service. There are also Medicare-sponsored educators who provide programs to demystify the various aspects of Medicare Parts A, B, D.

- Medicaid. Refer to your state's Medicaid website for specific details about this state and federal program.

- Health insurance. Do you have adequate health care coverage for yourself and your family?

- Life insurance. Have you discussed the advisability of purchasing life insurance with an insurance expert?

- Property tax–relief options. There are tax-relief programs available for low-income homeowners. Contact a real estate specialist or your local area agency on aging to determine the available programs in your area.

- Reverse mortgages. This is a financial vehicle that allows people sixty-two years of age and older to access the equity in their homes. Reverse mortgage specialists can provide the needed information to thoroughly evaluate this type of mortgage.

- Low-income home energy assistance program (LIHEAP). LIHEAP assists low-income people and families with utility expenses. For people on fixed incomes (i.e., retired people), this financial assistance is needed during the winter and summer seasons (times of extreme temperatures).

- Local and national foundations (respite care funding). Several disease-specific agencies and local foundations offer funds for respite care. Call your local area agency on aging to determine what programs are available in your area.

that could possibly happen as we age. But I can tell you that isolation and advanced age are rarely a good combination. Therefore, it is safe to assume that we will need easy access to personal, professional, community, and financial resources as we age. So plan accordingly. Position yourself such that you have access to that which you might need and want. By so doing, you can avoid the heartache and grief of Henry and Carmen.

So your mission is this (if you choose to accept it). Dream *big*! Your dream needs to include not only current but also future needs and desires. Utilize the SALAD approach to initially assess abilities and disabilities. Establish goals of care predicated on the needs and wants of the person. Develop, document, and implement a plan of care based on the available resources: personal, professional, community based, and financial. Then, as needs change, appropriately revise the goals and plan of care. Remember, to maintain a healthy plan, you'll need more than one SALAD. Life is ever changing. You must toss things around from time to time!

To Summarize...

🔍 The last step in the SALAD process is the development, documentation, and implementation of a plan of care. Obviously, the goals of care drive the plan of care. However, circumstances may preclude access to needed or desired resources to achieve a particular goal of care. The plan of care must be rooted in reality. If the available resources don't meet your needs and/or wants, it's time to tweak your plan.

🔍 In order to age well in place, we must plan well. Planning includes a proactive approach to aging and potential illness. By positioning ourselves in favorable locations, we will have access to the needed and desired resources as our care requirements change and increase. Access to services facilitates the development of an effective plan of care.

🔍 Do not become complacent once you have "tossed" a SALAD. With every change, positive or negative, the process of assessment, goal setting, and plan development must be revisited. You need to become adept at "tossing" a SALAD.

Chapter 11

Hospice and Palliative Care: Part of the Plan

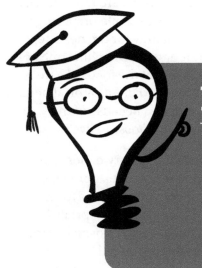

In This Chapter...

- What are hospice and palliative care?
- What is the history of hospice and palliative care?
- Why is hospice care important for patients and their families?
- How do hospice and palliative care work?

Creating a collaborative, compassionate, comprehensive plan of care is no small feat. In **Chapters 8–10**, we explored the healthy approach to assessment, goal generation, and plan development—SALAD. SALAD is a recipe for successfully evaluating and meeting the caregiving needs for family, friends, and ourselves. There are so many unknowns when attempting to anticipate future caregiving needs associated with progressive illness and advancing age. However, there is one given; we will all die. So, the pièce de résistance for a comprehensive plan of care is end-of-life planning.

Hospice and palliative care are philosophies of care, as well as models of care, that you need to understand. Ignorance regarding both models of care generates debilitating fear that serves to deter utilization of the needed and beneficial models of care. Not a surprising situation when you consider the depth and breadth of our societal aversion to death and dying. Please realize, we are not a death-*denying* society. How could we be? We are inundated with images of death on a daily basis via technology (television, Internet, and movies). However, we are a death-*averse* society. We disdain discussing death and the implications of our finitude. Technology serves to distance us from death as well. Few people know what death smells like, feels like, looks like, and sounds like. It is the intimacy of death that scares us. We don't know what to expect! Hospice and palliative care are approaches to care that address the immediate needs while preparing the patient and the family for the next step. When you understand the philosophy of care, you realize that the focus of care is on how we choose to *live* as mortal beings. Yes, we will die. And because of that reality, how do we *choose* to live?

After exploring the history of hospice and palliative care, we'll examine the particulars of both approaches to care. When is palliative care appropriate? How does a person enter hospice care? Who pays for the service? These and other questions will be answered, thus providing you with all the information necessary to make an informed decision around end-of-life care.

> ## Hospice and Palliative Care
>
> Palliative care is an interdisciplinary approach to medical care focused on enhancing the quality of life for those challenged by advanced illness.
>
> Hospice care is a type of palliative care reserved for those persons with terminal illness who have less than six months to live.
>
> **Definition**

Hospice and Palliative Care

Hospice and palliative care. Terms I'm sure you've heard before. I'm equally certain the terms are an enigma, unless you work in the field. Over the past ten years, I worked to demystify the concepts of hospice and palliative care. The commonly known myths about hospice serve to frighten the general population, reducing the utilization of this beneficial service. Palliative care is less frightening, but perhaps more confusing. So, let's begin at the beginning—definitions.

Palliative Care

Palliative care is a philosophy of care that recognizes cure is not always possible, but care always is. The Latin root, *palliare*, means to cloak or to shield. To palliate means to reduce the intensity of something or to alleviate symptoms without curing. Hence, the intent of palliative care is to shield or cloak patients from pain and suffering. The palliative care approach:

- recognizes that illness is a family challenge;

- expertly manages pain and symptoms;

- collaboratively generates goals of care;

- addresses the need for advance directives;

- optimizes the quality of life by anticipating, preventing, and treating suffering;

- coordinates care;

- addresses physical, emotional, cognitive, and spiritual aspects of care.

Palliative care is a specialized approach to care for persons with serious, chronic, or terminal illnesses. Curative treatments combined with palliative measures ensure the holistic care of the patient and the family. It is not enough to merely treat an illness. Palliative care serves the person—mind, body, and spirit. With a focus on the alleviation, anticipation, and prevention of suffering, palliative care enhances the quality of life for all involved. Interdisciplinary teams of health care professionals work collaboratively to address the physical, cognitive, emotional, spiritual, and psychosocial needs of the patient and family. Goals of care are identified. A plan of care developed. Coordination of care initiated. The palliative care teams typically include doctors, nurses, social workers, and chaplains.

Imagine someone in your family is diagnosed with ALS (Lou Gehrig's disease). ALS is not curable. As the illness progresses, pain and symptom

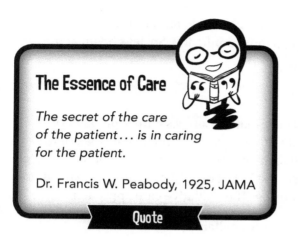

The Essence of Care

The secret of the care of the patient... is in caring for the patient.

Dr. Francis W. Peabody, 1925, JAMA

Quote

management becomes of paramount importance. Cure is not possible. But care is certainly needed and desired. Palliative care would be a tremendous benefit for your loved one and your family immediately following diagnosis. The palliative care team would help your family understand the disease process, treatment options, and prognosis. The team would listen to your concerns, your hopes, and your fears. Then the team would work collaboratively with your family to establish goals of care. This is incredibly important! The palliative care team isn't *telling* you what to do. Instead, the team strives to understand what is important to you. What constitutes an acceptable quality of life for the patient and the family? After defining the goals, the plan of care emerges and is implemented. Sound familiar? Well, it should. SALAD, our healthy approach to developing an effective plan of care for your family, mimics the palliative care approach: schedule, ask, listen, assess, and develop and implement. You know more about palliative care than you thought!

Hospice Care

Now that you have a foundational understanding of palliative care, let's consider hospice care. The philosophy of care is the same. Although cure is not possible, care is. *Hospice* is a type of palliative care focused on the care of the terminally ill. In the United States, persons deemed to have less than six months to live are eligible for hospice care. Unlike palliative care, hospice requires the termination of all curative measures for admittance. Hospice utilizes interdisciplinary teams as well. Later in the chapter, we will explore the detailed services provided by hospice. But for now, the main distinction between hospice and palliative care is this. To enroll in hospice, you must have a terminal diagnosis with an expectation of less than six months to live. You must also cease all curative treatments. As you might imagine, the requirement to stop curative treatments is a deterrent for some to enroll in hospice.

Don't Be Afraid

When asked to explain hospice and palliative care, I never attempt to "sell" the services to patients or families. Rather, I want people to choose the option of hospice and palliative care because they recognize the benefits of the service. In fact, I don't mention the word "hospice" when initially meeting with a family. "Hospice" prompts the same reaction as "cancer." People immediately stop listening. Their eyes glaze over. And they stare at the floor. There is no hope for a productive conversation when that happens. Fear just entered the room and derailed the process. I am better served if I go into the meeting "asking" instead of "telling." Once I know the lay of the land, I know how to introduce the idea of hospice and palliative care.

So I first need to understand the hopes and the fears of the patient and family. I don't presume to know your hopes and fears. But based on numerous studies as well as my experience with hospice families, there are some consistent themes. At the end of life, people typically want:

- effective pain and symptom management;

- a sense of control;

- to strengthen and/or reconcile relationships;

- to be home.

At the end of life, people typically fear:

- dying alone;

- being hooked up to machines;

- a prolonged death;

- dying in an institution;

- losing control (cognitively and physically);

- uncontrolled pain and symptoms;

- being a burden on the family.

I would imagine that you resonate with many of these hopes and fears. Assuming you do, what would you say if I told you there is a service that can minimize your fears? In fact, this same service enables you to achieve your hopes! If you are afraid of uncontrolled pain, I have a service that can help. If you want to die at home, I've got you covered there as well. You don't want to die alone? I can make sure that doesn't happen. How? Hospice and palliative care.

Example

Hospice—Thank Goodness!

I arrived early to my initial meeting with Mrs. Lewis. I wanted the time to review her charts. She was admitted to hospice earlier in the week with a diagnosis of metastatic lung cancer. Age eighty-five. As I entered the house, I met Mrs. Lewis' daughter and son. Mrs. Lewis was in her bedroom, unable to ambulate at this point. I was there to serve the entire family, so I spent some time listening to the children's concerns, answering questions, and providing some much-needed support. At the conclusion of our conversation, the family made a request. They asked that I remove my hospice badge. They didn't want their mother to know I was with hospice. They didn't want her to think they had given up. This was not the first time I had received such a request. Although I understood the "why" of the request, it always made me feel disingenuous. So I offered to take off my badge, but I told the family I would not lie to Mrs. Lewis. If she asked who I was and why I was there, I would tell her.

Mrs. Lewis was awake when I entered the room. Although she was physically frail, she was alert and coherent. I introduced myself, leaving out the fact that I worked for hospice. She looked directly at me and said, "You are with hospice, right?" Without hesitation, I said yes. She immediately smiled. Threw up her hands in celebration. "Thank goodness! I desperately need someone to talk to about what's happening. My children are scared to death I'm going to die. Too scared to talk about it. And I really need to talk about this. Before it's too late." And so we talked, well into the night.

Hospice is not to be feared. Hospice is a blessing to one and all.

To be honest, when I get to this point in the conversation, it doesn't matter what I call the service. The patient and the family *want* the service because they now see the benefits of this type of care. No selling required. When the benefits are known (education), hospice becomes the preferred choice of care at the end of life. Hospice and palliative care transform the lived experience of patients and families confronted by the challenges of chronic and/or terminal illness. These services are not to be feared. Rather, the services should be requested and embraced when the need arises.

Historical Development of Hospice and Palliative Care

Although hospice is a relatively new model of care in the United States, hospices have been around since the eleventh century. Originally, hospices were places where weary travelers could rest and recover. Today, the introduction and subsequent growth of hospice care is due in large part to three pioneers in end-of-life care. First, Dame Cecily Saunders established the first modern hospice in the United Kingdom in 1967. St. Christopher's Hospice served as the training ground and inspiration for other countries. Second, Elisabeth Kubler-Ross published her groundbreaking book, *On Death and Dying*, in 1969. This classic text explored the journey of dying from the perspective of the terminally ill patient. Kubler-Ross invited the world to discuss and debate a previously taboo subject—death and dying. Third, Florence Wald, a nurse from the United States, traveled to the United Kingdom to learn the hospice model of care under the tutelage of Saunders. Wald returned to Connecticut in 1974, where she opened the first hospice in the United States. These three women paved the way for enlightened discussions around patient care at the end of life. Their collective work and service contributed, in no small way, to the passage of the 1982 Medicare hospice benefit. Death and dying were front and center in Washington, DC. However, I am sure there were some congressional types stubbornly clinging to their immortal status. Some things never change!

Today, there are over 5,300 hospice organizations in the United States. According to the National Hospice and Palliative Care Organization, 1.65 million people received hospice care in 2011. Additionally, almost 45 percent of all deaths in the United States in 2011 occurred while in hospice. Although this figure is significant, the median length of service is only nineteen days. This means that people are entering hospice care very late in the disease

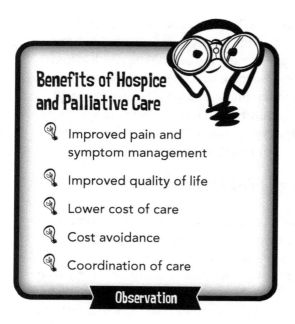

Benefits of Hospice and Palliative Care

- 🔍 Improved pain and symptom management
- 🔍 Improved quality of life
- 🔍 Lower cost of care
- 🔍 Cost avoidance
- 🔍 Coordination of care

Observation

process and thereby not receiving the full benefit of hospice care. We'll discuss the reasons for late admissions in the next section.

Dr. Balfour Mount is credited with coining the term palliative care. In 1975, he established the first palliative care program at the Royal Victoria Hospital in Montreal. In 1987, the Cleveland Clinic developed the first palliative care program in the United States. Then in 2006, hospice and palliative care was recognized as a subspecialty by the American Board of Medical Specialties. We have come a long way since Kubler-Ross initiated the needed discussions about death and dying. But we still have a long way to go in advancing the knowledge and subsequent utilization of hospice and palliative care.

The Benefits and Blessings of Hospice

Now that we understand the overarching philosophy of palliative care (which includes hospice care), let's discuss the specific benefits of hospice care. We can highlight many of the benefits by first dispelling the common myths about hospice. Following are some of the common myths regarding hospice:

- 🔍 *Myth—hospice is a place.* Many people fear they will have to relocate their loved one to a hospice facility. Although some larger hospices do have care centers, the majority of hospice care occurs in the home of the patient. This could be a house, apartment, or long-term care community. The hospice team comes to you. So one of the "hopes" noted previously is achieved through hospice care. You get to stay home!

- 🔍 *Myth—hospice provides only six months of care.* This myth causes late enrollment in hospice. People fear using up their benefit and then being discharged. This is *not* true! To enroll in hospice, a patient needs a doctor's order. The order indicates that based on the admitting condition, the doctor expects the person to die in less than six months. Once admitted, the hospice is required by Medicare to recertify patients periodically. As long as the patient is deemed to be "hospice appropriate," the patient remains in hospice care. The hospice benefit is *not* limited to six months.

Myth—hospice means there is no hope. Hospice, by definition, means there is no hope for cure. The patient must have a terminal illness to enroll in hospice. However, hospice is *all* about hope! Hope that pain and symptoms will be well managed. Hope that the patient can stay at home. Hope that the patient will be with family and friends. Hope that the surviving family will be supported and sustained after the death of the patient. Hope that relationships can be reconciled before death. Hope that the family will not be burdened. Hope that death will not be unduly prolonged. Hope that the patient will not die alone. Suffice it to say, hospice is *all* about *hope*!

Myth—hospice is only for cancer patients. Initially, the majority of patients in hospice were cancer patients. However, the patient population is changing. More and more people will die of complications associated with chronic illness. The increased incidence of chronic illness and the terminal designation of Alzheimer's disease have dramatically impacted the types of diseases seen in hospice. Hence, less than 50 percent of all hospice patients have cancer. Other admitting diagnoses include dementia, heart disease, lung disease, and nonspecific illness.

Myth—it's not time yet. Many people think hospice is only for the last few days of life. Entering hospice with only a few days or few hours to live is of no benefit to the patient or the family. Hence, I encourage people to enter hospice as soon as possible to reap the full benefits of care.

Myth—once enrolled, you can't get out. Patients have the right to discontinue hospice services at any time.

Myth—you can't keep your doctor if you enter hospice. Many doctors work collaboratively with hospice staff.

🔖 *Myth—when entering hospice, **all** medical treatment ceases.* It is required that curative treatments end prior to enrollment in hospice. However, treatments administered with a palliative intent (pain and symptom management) are obviously allowed.

🔖 *Myth—hospice is only for the elderly.* Hospice serves people of all ages with terminal illness. The prognosis of less than six months applies to all ages.

If you flip back to the list of the common hopes and fears at the end of life, you'll realize that hospice care alleviates the noted fears while helping patients and families live into their hopes. Is your fear around hospice dissipating? If not, read on.

In addition to what has already been noted, I would like to emphasize a few more benefits and blessings of hospice care:

🔖 Medicare requires that hospice organizations provide thirteen months of bereavement support for the surviving family (however you define family). This support can be bereavement support groups, private counseling, and/or periodic calls.

🔖 The patient and family members receive support from the hospice team. Quite often, family members fear the dying process. Hospice professionals provide education and information about what to expect—physically, emotionally, and spiritually.

🔖 Hospice provides continuous home care for brief periods of time for management of severe pain and symptoms.

🔖 Inpatient respite care is available as well. Family caregivers needing a break can arrange for up to five days of inpatient care at approved facilities.

🔖 Some hospices have general inpatient care units available for patients needing 24/7 care. This is usually a short-term proposition; the patient is transferred back home once the issue is resolved.

There is much to be said about the benefits and blessings of hospice. If you have experience with hospice, personally or professionally, you can add to

The Hospice Difference

Hospice care was not available when my mom died in 1981. However, seventeen years later when my dad was suffering from metastatic prostate cancer, hospice cared for our family. I remember the first meeting with the hospice admissions nurse. I was clueless and somewhat confused. Hospice was a foreign concept. The hospice nurse patiently explained how hospice would care for my dad and for our family. At the time, my brother and I both lived out of state. So news of additional help was greatly appreciated.

As I compare the end-of-life journey with my mom with that of my dad, there is no comparison. Quite often with my mom, I felt afraid, isolated, and frustrated. There were so many unknowns. And the unknowns generated a tremendous amount of fear and anxiety. With my dad, hospice served to educate, to guide, and to support all of us. Hospice enabled us to be present to the moment, to spend sacred time together as a family. It was an amazing gift, one I wish we could have shared with my mom as well.

Observation

the list. Having experienced the death of my mom without hospice and the death of my dad with hospice, I know the benefits of hospice from the inside out.

Nuts and Bolts of Hospice Care

If you started this chapter fearing hospice, you should know enough by now to at least be curious instead of frightened. You have the foundational information about this model of care: definition, philosophy of care, historical development, and benefits of care. Perhaps now you are interested in the logistical aspects of hospice: enrollment, payment, and specific services.

How Do You Enroll in Hospice?

Many people assume that if and when hospice care is appropriate, the doctor will initiate the discussion of end-of-life care. If you don't remember anything else from this chapter, please remember this. Be your own best advocate for end-of-life care. Do not assume your doctor will broach the subject. *Do not wait.* Ask the question. Is it time for hospice? If your doctor ignores the question, refuses to discuss end-of-life options, or discounts the benefits of hospice care, I strongly recommend that you seek a second opinion. In order to enroll in hospice, you must have a doctor's order indicating the terminal nature of your illness and confirming a prognosis of less than six months to live. Some doctors are reluctant to refer patients to hospice, viewing this referral as a professional failure. The doctor failed to cure, and cure is what medical schools train doctors to do. That is the expectation. So instead of referring to hospice, many doctors continue to push curative measures. This culture of "cure at all costs" is changing. However, you may still encounter resistance within the medical community.

When considering enrollment into hospice care, you have the right to select a hospice. I encourage people to interview hospices just like you would any another medical service provider. Seek recommendations. Call and talk to the admissions staff. Get a feel for how the organization interacts with the patients and families. All hospices provide the same basic services mandated by the Medicare hospice benefit. That is not the issue. Rather, you need to find a hospice that "feels" right for you and your family. This is an important decision. Take the time to explore your options.

Who Pays for Hospice?

Hospice is a Medicare benefit reimbursed on a per diem (per day) basis. Every day a person is in hospice care, the provider gets reimbursed a predetermined amount of money. The rates of reimbursement change periodically. However, to give you an idea of the fee structure, these were the rates through September 2013:

- Routine care (in home): $153.45/day

- Continuous home care: $895.56/day

- Inpatient respite care: $158.72/day

- General inpatient care: $682.59/day

Who pays for hospice care? Medicare (Part A), Medicaid, private insurance, and

Ask for Hospice— Don't Wait for an Invitation

Doctors are trained in the medical model of care. As such, they are trained to cure. Now don't misunderstand. I am quite thankful my doctor is intent on curing me. However, there will come a time in my life when cure is not possible. When that time comes, I want my doctor to have the courage and the ability to have "the" conversation with me. I want to discuss the option of palliative and hospice care. If, by chance, my doctor misses the opportunity to initiate the conversation, I won't be shy. I will ask for the care I want and need.

IMPORTANT!

private pay. Additionally, some hospices underwrite the care of those unable to pay for services.

What Does Hospice Care Include?

Hospice care includes the following:

- Medications for the terminal condition. Medications for other conditions or illnesses are not covered by the hospice benefit.

- Medical equipment. Equipment listed in the written plan of care is included. Items could include hospital beds, bedside commode, shower chairs, etc.

- Staff. Doctors, nurses, CNAs, social workers, chaplains, administrative staff, pharmacists, bereavement specialists, and volunteers. Routine hospice care does not consist of 24/7 staff in the home. The hospice team schedules visits based on the specific needs of the patient. If needed, hospice can be contacted 24/7 to address questions and concerns.

- Medical supplies. Things such as dressings, syringes, etc.

- Alternative therapies. Complementary therapies are not required by Medicare. However, larger hospice organizations often offer services such as music therapy, art therapy, animal-assisted therapy, massage, and aromatherapy.

- Bereavement services. Medicare requires that hospice organizations provide thirteen months of bereavement services for family members.

Nuts and Bolts of Palliative Care

As a former palliative care educator, I presented programs singing the praises of the philosophy of palliative care. This was an easy song to sing since I truly believe this is the humane approach to practicing medicine. I would compare and contrast hospice and palliative care, explaining that palliative care is not limited to terminal illness or end-of-life care. In the case of serious or chronic illness, the goal of palliative care is to enhance the quality of life for the patient and family. An admirable goal, one that caught the attention of many people who have heard me speak. Without fail, at least one person would ask how they could enroll their mother or father in palliative care. Or could I recommend a palliative care doctor? And, without fail, I always felt as if I had set people up for disappointment. The old carrot and stick routine. I dangled the carrot of palliative care. Shed light on a different approach to medical care. Convinced people that palliative care is the compassionate approach to care. And then, I had to tell them access to palliative care services is limited. Sorry! Here comes the stick, right?

If palliative care is such a fabulous model of care, why are services limited? Money. Plain and simple. Unlike hospice, palliative care services are not fully reimbursed by Medicare and Medicaid. Private insurance and HMOs *may* cover certain aspects of palliative care, but you need to check with your provider. Until the reimbursement structure changes, access to palliative care will be limited.

Access to Palliative Care

Access to palliative care will remain limited in the United States without revision of the current reimbursement provisions.

Observation

Currently, palliative care is provided in hospitals, hospices, long-term care communities, and home settings. The predominant model of service is the hospital-based consultation service. If you are in the hospital, you might be eligible for a palliative care consult. A palliative care team or a solo practitioner meets with you and your family to discuss your situation. Goals of care are established. A plan of care is created. Care is coordinated. However, upon discharge, you may or may not be "followed home" by palliative care services. Consequently, there is oftentimes a lack of follow-through and follow-up with care receivers and family members.

Many hospices offer palliative care services, as evidenced by the name of the organization: ABC Hospice and Palliative Care. There are a couple reasons for this. As we noted earlier, many people are afraid of hospice, the word "hospice." Consequently, the person will decline hospice care but might agree to palliative care. Once enrolled, the person may or may not transition over to hospice care. Even though palliative care programs are an expense, many organizations use the palliative care program as a marketing tool for the hospice program. As a palliative care patient transitions to hospice care, the provider benefits by an increase in its hospice census.

So where can you get palliative care? Well, it depends! It depends on where you live. Are there palliative care providers in the area? Depends on what you can afford. Palliative care is not fully reimbursed. And it depends on your diagnosis. There are some managed-care organizations that offer disease-specific palliative care services. For example, cancer, congestive heart failure, or ALS (Lou Gehrig's Disease) qualify for a palliative care consult. MS may not. Again, you need to explore the specifics with your provider.

We will no doubt witness the continuing evolution of palliative care in the years to come. Demographic changes necessitate changes in medical services and systems. Things will change! Stating the obvious, right? My personal hope for palliative care is this. I hope palliative care becomes the standard of care, the expectation for *all* clinicians. This isn't an unrealistic expectation if you understand the basic tenets of palliative care. Is it too much to ask of our doctors to communicate effectively with the patient *and* the family? Is it unreasonable to expect our doctors to be adept at managing symptoms and pain? Is it too lofty an expectation to be served as a person instead of treated as an illness? And is it absurd to think the patient and family should have a voice in designing a plan of care? These are not unreasonable expectations. My fervent hope is that this becomes the reality in the very near future. You and I will be well served when palliative care is the norm.

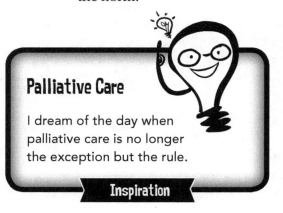

Palliative Care

I dream of the day when palliative care is no longer the exception but the rule.

Inspiration

Hospice Is Transformational

As part of my seminary training, I opted to enroll in Clinical Pastoral Education (CPE). CPE entails a clinical placement (hospital, faith community, hospice) and associated classes. I explored a variety of placement options, subconsciously discounting the option of hospice. At that time, I couldn't imagine companioning terminally ill patients and their families. It struck too close to the bone. Hospice threatened to trigger unpleasant memories of my mom's death and shed light on my hidden grief. I wasn't ready to feel that exposed, that raw. Well, ready or not, that's what happened! Long story short, I served as a hospice chaplain intern for a year. Upon completion of my internship, I served as the Director of Education for a palliative care educational institute for six years. During my tenure, I felt exposed, raw, *and* alive. My professional experience of hospice changed my life, changed my perception of life and death. So, my friends, *fear not*! Hospice and palliative care can, and will, serve you and yours well when the need arises. Consequently, hospice and palliative care are essential ingredients for your comprehensive plan of care.

To Summarize...

- An essential ingredient in a plan of care is end-of-life planning. Hospice and palliative care services provide support and care for patients and families challenged by serious and terminal illness. Do not let your fear of death and dying inhibit your ability to access the care you need at the end of life. Learn what hospice and palliative care services have to offer. Then integrate the end-of-life services into your comprehensive plan of care.

- Palliative care is a philosophy of care focused on enhancing the quality of life for those persons and families challenged by serious illness. Even if cure is not possible, care always is. Hospice is a type of palliative care reserved for those persons diagnosed with a terminal illness, expected to live less than six months.

- We need to be our own best advocates when it comes to medical care. Do not wait to be invited to discuss the option of palliative and/or hospice care. When confronted with a serious, chronic, or terminal illness, talk with your doctor about the advisability and the availability of palliative and hospice care. You need to know your options in order to make the best decisions for you and your loved ones.

- Hospice is a Medicare benefit (Part A) that requires a doctor's order for enrollment. Typical payers of hospice care include Medicare, Medicaid, private insurance, and private pay. Palliative care is only partially reimbursed through Medicare, Medicaid, and private insurance.

Chapter 12

Plan for Life!

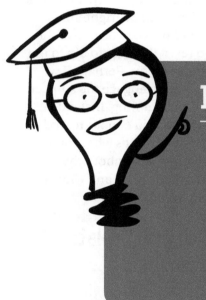

In This Chapter...

- Will your wishes equal your reality at the end of life?

- What stops you from having the needed conversation with family and friends about *life?*

- What are the options for documenting your wishes for *life?*

- Why should you Plan for *Life?*

Planning is hard work, isn't it? If Boomers are to age *well*, we must plan well! In the last four chapters, I've encouraged you to embrace and to employ the recipe for successful planning. SALAD: Schedule, Ask, Listen, Assess, and Develop. If you are the type of cook who strictly adheres to the recipe, you may think you're done. Well, think again. I always throw in something extra on my salads. Croutons. Grated cheese. Something! When preparing to care, the little something extra is advance directives.

Advance directives are legal documents that indicate your preferences related to medical care and end-of-life care. These documents become effective if you are incapacitated or are unable to speak for yourself. This could be due to an accident, illness, or advanced age. You might be twenty-two or ninety-three. If you are of legal age, you should seriously consider identifying, articulating, and documenting your wishes. If not for you, then for your family. Although I will review the various forms, my focus is on the conversations needed to convey your wishes to family and friends. In order to speak for you, they must *know* you. Not only know what you *want*, but know who you *are*. Our wants change, but our essence abides.

I invite you to open your mind and heart to the topic of advance directives. I realize this is not the hot topic on a Friday night! It can be frightening, confusing, emotional, and distressing. But it could prove to be one of the most important ingredients in your SALAD. So resist the urge to flip to the next chapter. I have some ideas to "toss" around with you. Perhaps if we reframe the discussion, you might be more inclined to engage the subject. Don't think about this as the traditional end-of-life planning. Instead, contemplate how you choose to *live*! Because, in reality, that's what you're doing. So start thinking about the who, what, when, where, how, and why *before* you die! Plan for *Life*!

Advance Directives

Legal documents that indicate your preferences for medical care and end-of-life care. The documents become effective if you are incapacitated and/or are unable to articulate your preferences.

Definition

Motivation to Articulate Your Wishes

Over the past ten years, I have addressed the issue of advance directives with individuals, families, and audiences. Believe me, I know this subject is not number one on the hit parade! However, advance directives are an incredibly important ingredient in your plan of care. If omitted, your carefully conceived plan of care contains a fatal flaw. You have not determined how you wish the plan to end. How would you prefer to conclude your journey? Granted, there are things beyond your control, things you'll fail to anticipate. But considering the "what ifs" is part of the process, an important part.

Let's consider some "what ifs." The following scenarios describe very common situations in health care today. Common, but extraordinarily difficult for the ill-prepared and ill-equipped family. So what would you do in these what-if scenarios?

The doctor just concluded a review of your mother's condition. Not good. She is in the late stage of Alzheimer's disease, so not surprising. But hearing the details of her condition is distressing. This is the day your family has been dreading. Your mother is no longer able to swallow. So the doctor posed the question of artificial nutrition and hydration. Do you know what your mother wants? Is your family in agreement as to how to proceed? Are your mother's wishes documented? What will you do?

Since being diagnosed with ALS (Lou Gehrig's disease) several years ago, you and your family have worked as a team to make the best of a very bad situation. Today, your team is conflicted about the next step in the journey, the step of ventilation. Your doctor provided the needed information, answered questions, and explained the reality of the situation. Your family, your team, wants you to agree to ventilation. They are not ready to say goodbye. But you are. What will you do?

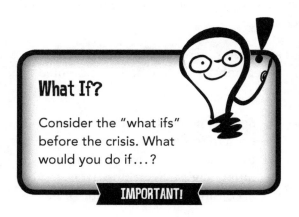

What If?

Consider the "what ifs" before the crisis. What would you do if . . . ?

IMPORTANT!

The ER doctor called ten minutes ago. Your husband was involved in a horrific accident. Head trauma. Life support. Little hope. These are the phrases you remember from the call. *This isn't happening! He's only forty-seven years old. We are supposed to get old and gray together. What would he want? Why didn't we talk about this before? Why do I have to make the decision?* These and a thousand other questions confuse and confound you on the way to the emergency room. What will you do?

Life happens, doesn't it? And not always as planned. However, if you are to have *any* say in the matter, you must convey your wishes to your family and health care providers. This process begins with self-reflection, identifying what it is you want and don't want. Know thyself. Once you've identified your wishes, talk to your family. Document your wishes using the various forms available. Then provide copies of the documents to everyone involved with your care: family, friends, health care providers. If you wish to be in control, you should *love* the premise of advance directives. Even when you are incapacitated and unable to speak for yourself, you are still directing traffic. Since I am a professed control queen, I find this thought very comforting!

You are in good company if you have not completed your advance directives. "Good" indicating a large number of people, not "good on you!" Recent surveys document the fact that what we wish for is not what we experience at the end of life. Perhaps a few statistics will motivate you and your family to initiate the process. As the numbers reveal, what we want and what we get are dramatically different. According to a report published in 2012 by the California HealthCare Foundation:

- Sixty percent of those surveyed don't want their families forced to make tough decisions at end of life. However, 56 percent of those surveyed had *not* discussed their wishes with family members.

- Eighty percent of those surveyed wanted to discuss end-of-life options with their health care provider. Only 7 percent surveyed had discussed their wishes with their doctor.

- Eighty-two percent of those surveyed said documentation of end-of-life wishes is important. However, only 23 percent had documented their wishes.

- Seventy percent of those surveyed want to receive care in the home, to die at home. However, 70 percent ultimately die in facilities (this according to the Centers for Disease Control, 2005).

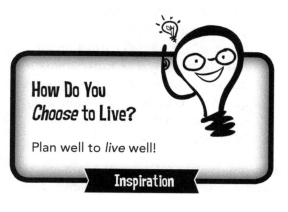

How Do You Choose to Live?

Plan well to *live* well!

Inspiration

Now, I will be the first one to admit that advance directives are not 100 percent foolproof and airtight. For a variety of reasons, advance directives may be ignored, changed, or discounted. Even so, the process of identifying, articulating, and documenting your wishes is worthwhile—for you and your family. By doing so, you increase the odds that your end-of-life wishes will equal your reality.

Barriers to Advance Care Planning

Depending on the source of information, it is estimated that only 25 to 30 percent of the population in the United States have advance directives in place. Why do most people omit this important ingredient from the plan of care? There are a variety of reasons, but these are the ones I hear most often:

- Advance who? Some people neglect to identify, articulate, and document their wishes due to ignorance of the process. If the need is not recognized, the person has no motivation to act.

- Not old enough. Youth provides a false sense of security. If you are of legal age, you need to consider completing advance directives. We have far too many examples of people in the prime of life tragically compromised by illness or accident. Without advance directives, the families were left to make the tough decisions, often debating the merits of various options in court. If of legal age, it is never too soon to identify, articulate, and document your wishes.

- Fear of death and dying. Many people avoid the discussion of end-of-life care due to an overwhelming fear of death and dying. They can't or won't go there. The fear of the unknown is paralyzing. Or perhaps the fear is predicated on a previous experience of death within the family. Those who have witnessed tremendous suffering and difficult deaths will do one of two things. Either they will enthusiastically engage the process to ensure they will not experience the same fate or they will avoid the subject altogether.

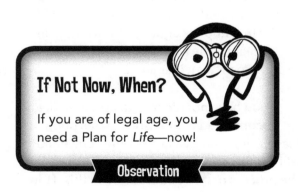

If Not Now, When?

If you are of legal age, you need a Plan for *Life*—now!

Observation

Distrust of the medical system. Based on historical events, a person or group of people may have an inherent distrust of the health care system. Advance directives are perceived as an extension of "the system" and are, therefore, not to be trusted.

Culturally inappropriate. In some cultures, end-of-life care is deemed the responsibility of the family. As such, the family will naturally make all needed decisions. No documentation is needed, wanted, or required.

Emotionally too hard. For some people, it is too emotionally distressing to consider end-of-life concerns. Usually the emotions are a manifestation of a significant fear of death and dying. By recognizing and honoring the emotions, you can then deal with the source of the resistance, fear.

Family dissension. Perhaps you are ready to sit down with your family and discuss your end-of-life wishes. But your family isn't! Where do you go from there? Later in the chapter, we will discuss some different approaches to starting the conversation. Timing is critically important. Are you in the middle of a crisis? Or are you proactively planning for your ultimate demise? Make sure the timing is such that your family is able and willing to engage the topic. Additionally, *how* you extend the invitation is equally important. This is meant to be a collaborative process. Be sure to present it as such.

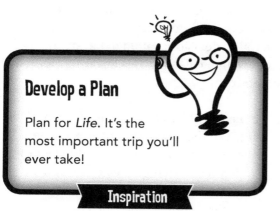

Develop a Plan

Plan for *Life*. It's the most important trip you'll ever take!

Inspiration

If you have not identified, articulated, and documented your wishes to this point, it is important to understand the reasons for your hesitation or procrastination. Remember, knowledge is power. From that position, you can make an informed decision to complete the process or not. Let me ask you this. How much time did you spend planning a vacation this year? How much time and effort have you invested in your financial plan? If you have children, have you explored and planned for the possibility of college? My point being, we are planners (some better, some worse). We establish a goal (vacation, retirement, college), and we make plans to achieve that goal. Pretty simple. The same is true for the last leg of the journey. Establish goals. Make a plan. Voila! Wishes equal reality. To assume that things will "just fall into place" is to risk seeing your life fall apart well before the finish line. I encourage you to plan well in order to finish strong. Plan for *Life*!

Identify Your Wishes

Before you can *articulate* and *document* your wishes for *life*, you must first *identify* your wishes. What is of greatest importance to you? What enhances the quality of your *life*? What aspects are essential? What are optional? This is the kind of self-reflection needed to Plan for *Life*. When creating your Plan for *Life*, access the resources needed to make the best plan possible. Speak with your doctor about treatment options. Talk to your family. Chat with your friends. Debate. Discuss. Encourage. Explore. Collaboration enriches and enhances the planning process.

During this time of self-reflection and discussion, you begin to realize that your wishes for *life* are a consequence of your hopes and fear. For example, if you fear experiencing uncontrollable pain, you will wish for effective pain and symptom management. So, one way to identify your wishes for *life* is to first list your hopes and fears.

What are your hopes? (Generate your own list.)

- Remain at home.

- Be surrounded by family, friends, and critters.

- Retain a sense of control.

- Be treated with dignity and respect.

- Receive compassionate care.

- Experience well-managed pain and symptoms.

What are your fears? (Generate your own list.)

- Loss of control

- Loss of relationships

- Loss of dignity

- Being a burden

- Loss of meaning and purpose

Pure Genius!

Dinner and Directives

Discussing our wishes for medical care and end-of-life care need not be morbid. Consider this idea. A man in his early thirties had a near miss on the ski slopes of Colorado. On the drive down from the mountains that night, he wondered who would have been there for him *if* he had ended up in the ER. The thought rattled him since he had no answer. So, the following week, he invited five of his best friends over for a lovely meal. They enjoyed fabulous food, lovely wine, and lively conversation.

After dinner, the host initiated an amazing discussion. He thanked everyone for attending and sharing a lovely evening. This group was his family. The people he knew the best and loved the most! And because of that, he wanted to make sure that now and in the future, they could all take care of each other. He shared his story from the past weekend on the ski slopes. This experience shattered his illusion of control and immunity. He needed and wanted a plan. Furthermore, he wanted his friends to be a part of his plan.

Initially, the group was a bit tentative to "go there." However, as the conversation unfolded, every person at the table shared their hopes and fears. Every person eventually articulated wishes for *life*. And every person was heard, honored, and supported. Advance directives can be presented in creative, enticing ways! Food for thought, eh?

- Physical suffering

- Loss of home

- Financial ruin

Once you've identified your hopes and fears, you can now easily generate your wishes for *life*. I wish to stay home. I wish to have a voice in my plan of care. I wish to have my four cats on my bed at all times. Whatever supports, sustains, and serves you, wish it and make it so!

Articulating Your Wishes

Now that you have identified your wishes for *life*, it's time to articulate your wishes. Those who will be responsible for your care need to *hear* your *life* wishes, not just read them. As we all know, the written word can be misconstrued. You want no misunderstandings when it comes to your *life* wishes. Plus, you want to give your family the opportunity to ask questions, reflect, and clarify. This need not be a morbid, depressing discussion. You can be as innovative and creative as you choose.

Kick-Start the Conversation

Up to this point, I assumed you were the person needing and wanting a Plan for *Life*. When self-motivated, you can move through the process fairly quickly. But what if you are trying to motivate someone else to create a Plan for *Life*? And what if they are not *thrilled* about the idea? Remember the barriers for planning noted earlier in the chapter? You may have to overcome significant resistance. How you introduce the idea is very important. You don't want the process to end before you get started!

If you need some suggestions on how to kick-start the needed *life* conversations, I have a few ideas. Have you ever heard of Go Wish Cards? If not, check out this resource online (codaalliance.org). Go Wish Cards reflect the common hopes and fears related to the end-of-life experience. A deck consists of thirty-six cards. Each card indicates a common wish expressed by those confronted by a serious or terminal illness. For example, one of the wishes is "to be mentally aware." The cards are a fabulous way to invite your family to discuss some tough topics. Most people enjoy playing card games. So the cards are not intimidating. And you can make a game of it. Consider the following:

1. Invite your family over for lunch on Sunday afternoon.

2. After lunch, clear the table. Give everyone a deck of Go Wish Cards. You can purchase the cards online. Also, some hospices loan out the cards to community members.

3. Be honest about your objective. You want to understand what is important to each person sitting around your table in regard to how they *wish* to *live*. By knowing what is important, you can support them in their journey. And you want them to support you in yours. You can do that only if you know the wishes of the other person.

4. Using the cards, each person will identify his or her top five wishes for *life*.

5. First, read all the wishes on the cards. Then, divide the cards into three categories. Critical Wishes. Nice Wishes. Irrelevant Wishes.

6. Then, from the cards in the Critical Wishes group, select your top five wishes for *life*. Don't show them to anyone else at the table.

7. Once done, the conversation begins. Ask your family to guess the five cards you hold in your hands. The odds are, they won't guess all five correctly. That is when the conversation gets interesting. "Wow. I never knew that was important to you. Good to know!" Continue around the table until everyone has the opportunity to "lay their cards on the table."

8. This is a conversation your family will never forget. You may choose to have periodic "card games" since our *life* wishes change as we age.

There are two other resources that will assist in kick-starting the needed conversations in your family. First, *Caring Conversations* is a guide available through the Center for Practical Bioethics (practicalbioethics.org). Second, The Conversation Project (theconversationproject.org) provides information and strategies designed to facilitate the needed conversations as well. I am not married to any particular resource. Use what works best for you and your family. I don't care how you start talking. Just get started!

Documentation Options

It is now time to discuss your options for documenting your wishes. Advance directives is a term that refers to a number of different forms. Each form serves a particular purpose. Collectively, the forms serve to designate a health care agent, document health care instructions, and document other wishes. A comprehensive discussion of the forms is neither my intent nor my desire. Instead, I want to highlight how each form serves to ensure that your wishes become your reality. My comments are of a general nature, not specific to any one state. Hence, I encourage you to explore the specifics of your home state to ensure the efficacy of the forms chosen to document your wishes. With that disclaimer in place, let's look briefly at the basic forms available that serve to document your *life* wishes:

- Living will. A legal document that describes your wishes concerning life-sustaining treatments in the case of terminal illness or persistent vegetative state (PVS). The living will becomes effective when you are deemed incapacitated. Of importance to note, if you do not suffer from a terminal illness or PVS, the living will does not become effective.

- Medical durable power of attorney. A legal document that designates your health care agent, the person who will make medical decisions for you when incapacitated. Your agent is to act in accordance with your wishes and values. Choose your health care agent wisely. This is probably *the* most important element of your advance directives. We'll discuss health care agents specifically in the following section.

- CPR directive. Cardiopulmonary resuscitation directive is a legal form documenting your wish *not* to receive CPR if you experience cardiac or pulmonary arrest. This type of directive is typically used by terminally ill or elderly persons. CPRs require that both the patient and physician sign the order. A CPR differs from a DNR (do not resuscitate) in that DNRs are effective only while the patient is in a health care facility (including a nursing home).

Speaking for Aunt Jane

I served as the health care agent for my godmother, Aunt Jane. She didn't shrink from the reality of life. We shared many a pointed discussion as to what she wanted and what she didn't regarding medical care and end-of-life care. There was no doubt in my mind as to what her wishes were. So when the doctor called to discuss the option of a feeding tube for Aunt Jane, I knew exactly what to say. I said, "*No.*" That was Aunt Jane's wish, and I honored it. I also cried for hours after that call, knowing the consequences of that decision. Doing the right thing for those we love at the end of the journey is often the hardest thing we'll ever do in this life. Speaking for Aunt Jane was a sacred honor and an incredible challenge for me.

Example

MOST. Medical orders for scope of treatment is a relatively new form of advance directive. The form documents the patient's wishes for CPR, medical interventions, antibiotics, and artificial nutrition. When signed by both the physician and patient, the form becomes part of the medical orders and follows the patient even when transferred to another location.

POLST. Physician orders for life-sustaining treatment are the same as above, just a different name. Depends on the state in which you live which form is used.

Five Wishes. This is a form available through Aging with Dignity, a nonprofit organization. Due to its popularity throughout the country, I chose to note the form. The first wish is the designation of a health care agent. *The* most important wish. The remaining wishes address options for medical care, personal care, and final arrangements.

Once you have completed the forms, make copies for all persons involved in your Plan for *Life*. Your family, friends, and health care providers. It's also important to recognize the evolutionary nature of your Plan for *Life*. Your wishes will change as you age. What I wished for at twenty-five is quite different from what I wish for today. My view of life is different. My wants and needs are different. So my advance directives must reflect my current perspectives to serve me well. Consequently, I encourage you to review and update your Plan for *Life* every couple of years. This is an iterative process. Stay current.

Your Wish Is My Command

I realize the process of planning for *life* can be intimidating. You may have spent your entire life avoiding "the" conversation and the fun of filling out advance directive forms. If so, let me make this easier for you. If you don't do anything else, name a health care agent to speak for you when you can't. This is *the* most important piece of the puzzle. This is the person you literally trust with your life. The person who *knows* you, inside and out. The person with whom you've shared your hopes, fears, and wishes. The person whom you trust implicitly. And the person who agrees to do this for you. This is not an easy role to assume. In fact, it was one of the hardest things I have ever done.

There are legal stipulations as to who can serve as your health care agent, typically a person of legal age with decisional capacity. Your health care agent has the ability to accept or refuse treatment as well as request the withdrawal of treatment on your behalf. The decisions of your health care agent should be predicated on your directives and wishes.

When choosing your health care agent, choose wisely. You may opt to ask a trusted family member. Or you may realize that person will be emotionally distraught at the time of your demise. So perhaps it would be better to select a close friend. There is no one right answer. It just depends. My best advice is this. Your health care agent needs to be a pit bull. Tenacious. Courageous. Strong. Loyal. Fearless. Your health care agent needs a steely spine and the ability to confront family members, medical professionals, and possibly legal types if push comes to shove. Your health care agent must be able and willing to plead your case and fight your fight if necessary. This is not a role for the faint of heart. Once you decide, sit down with the person and explain exactly what you wish. Answer any questions. Address any concerns. If the person agrees to be your health care agent, you are blessed indeed. It takes a person of tremendous courage and conviction to walk with you to the end of the road.

One note of caution. If you are considering designating coagents, *don't*! You have the option to designate a primary, secondary, and tertiary agent in the event that your primary agent is incapable or unavailable to serve. This is a good idea. But designating two people to share the role of health care agent is a train wreck waiting to happen. What if the two people disagree as to what is in your best interest? In the extreme, this can lead to expensive, divisive court battles. Avoid this by designating one primary health care agent who is committed to serving you well. This will help ensure your wishes become your reality.

Ethical Wills

Ethical wills have little to do with your wishes regarding medical care and end-of-life care. However, I include the topic because ethical wills are a lovely, ancient tradition that should be included in our Plan for *Life*. As we are contemplating our mortality and planning how we choose to live until our very last breath, I think it important to contemplate the message, the legacy, we choose to leave for generations to come. A parting gift.

A Parting Note

One of the greatest gifts and blessings my dad bestowed on me was a letter. A letter I found after his death. It was in the middle drawer of his desk, waiting to be discovered. My brother and I had been boxing up our dad's personal effects when we came upon the letters. As I read the letter addressed to me, my heart overflowed. In the letter, my dad finally said the things I had longed to hear my entire life. And in many ways, I felt as if I finally knew my dad. A blessing indeed.

Inspiration

Ethical wills are nonbinding documents that reflect a person's values and beliefs. Blessings may be offered. Advice given to subsequent generations. The practice stems for the ancient Judeo-Christian tradition when ethical wills were conveyed orally. It is a lovely tradition, and one that is going through a resurgence of late. Perhaps it is because we realize the value of a person's life is not measured by the gold left behind. Instead, we are measured by the impact and the effect our life had on others. It is our story that is ultimately timeless and priceless.

The Gifts of Planning

So, have I convinced you? Are you a believer that planning for *life* is worthy of your time and attention? Is there merit to my premise that advance directives increase the odds that your wishes will become your reality? Well, if not, I have one more thing in my bag of goodies to

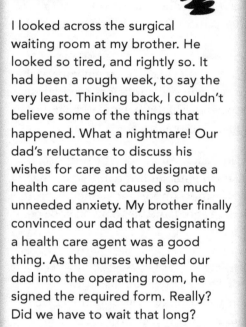

Racing Down the Hall

I looked across the surgical waiting room at my brother. He looked so tired, and rightly so. It had been a rough week, to say the very least. Thinking back, I couldn't believe some of the things that happened. What a nightmare! Our dad's reluctance to discuss his wishes for care and to designate a health care agent caused so much unneeded anxiety. My brother finally convinced our dad that designating a health care agent was a good thing. As the nurses wheeled our dad into the operating room, he signed the required form. Really? Did we have to wait that long?

Uninspired

entice you to Plan for *Life*. Do this for the people you love and who love you. Do this for your family! Believe me, I know the anxiety and stress your reluctance can potentially cause your family.

So remember, planning for *life* benefits you and your family in the following ways:

- Removes doubt. Your family knows what you want.

- Allows you to retain some control over what happens.

- Reduces the burden on your family. You made the decisions.

- Reduces (doesn't eliminate) family conflict and debate.

By identifying, articulating, and documenting your wishes, you added that little something extra to the SALAD process that makes all the difference. You officially added your thumbprint to the process identifying it as *yours*. Your wants, your needs, your desires, your goals, and your wishes. This is *your* Plan for *Life*. I hope it turns out exactly as you wished.

To Summarize...

Advance directive is a frightening and/or confusing term for most people. It's hard to get excited about legal forms and end-of-life planning. So I invite you to think about the process in a different way. Think about how you want to *live*, until your very last breath. Your Plan for *Life* is the little something extra needed for your SALAD. The finishing touch!

Your Plan for *Life* requires you to identify, articulate, and document your wishes for medical care and end-of-life care. Granted, you can't anticipate everything that could possibly happen over the course of your lifetime. However, your plan will increase the odds that your wishes equal your reality.

Advance directives include a variety of forms, each with a specific purpose. It is important to know what is legally recognized in your state and any state-specific stipulations related to advance directives. *The* most important element in your Plan for *Life* is the designation of a health care agent, the person who will speak for you when you are incapacitated.

Upon completion of your Plan for *Life*, provide copies of all documents to everyone involved with your care—family, friends, and health care providers. Remember, your Plan for *Life* will change as you change. Consequently, revisit your plans periodically and update as needed. Provide copies of the revised version to all involved.

Your Plan for *Life* is a tremendous gift to your family, friends, and yourself. Plan well and live well.

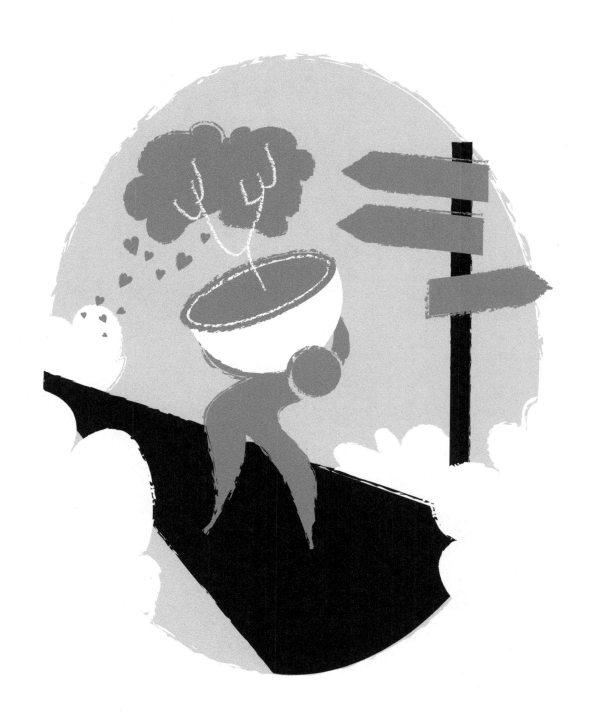

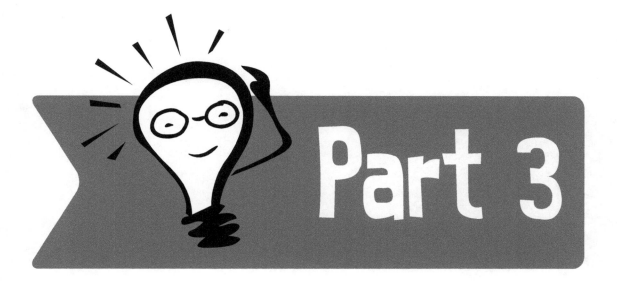

The Stressful Journey of Caregiving

It is now time for the mandatory discussion about caregivers and stress. We all know that caregiving is a stressful proposition, right? The various changes experienced throughout the journey of caregiving stress everyone involved. Caregiver and care receiver alike incur losses and, therefore, feel vulnerable and at risk. We feel exposed and overwhelmed. Preparing to care mitigates some of the stress of caregiving. However, stress cannot be entirely eliminated from the process. The challenge then becomes recognition and management of stress to minimize the risk of compromising our own health and well-being when serving as caregivers. So, be realistic about the caregiving journey. Caregiving is stressful. The key to handling the stress is to identify the sources of your stress, recognize how you manifest stress, and then effectively address your stress.

Chapter 13

Stressing Stress

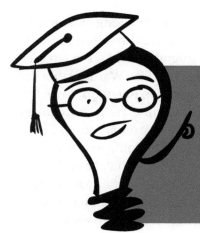

In This Chapter...

- What are the risks of being a caregiver?
- What factors serve to increase stress?
- How do we express our stress?

I have attended and presented many caregiving programs over the past ten years. Without fail, there is a portion of the program dedicated to the discussion of caregiver stress. I have yet to attend or present a program that does this topic justice. The journey of caregiving is stressful for the caregiver and the care receiver. Based on the specifics of the situation, stress is a consequence of a myriad of factors. So to address the stress appropriately and effectively requires a foundational understanding of the source of the stress.

What do I mean by stress? Stress is defined as our response to stressors (real or imagined) that disrupts our physical or mental equilibrium. In simplistic terms, a pebble falls into our pond of tranquility, resulting in ripples or possibly waves (depending on the size of the pebble). Our world is rocked for a period of time until the desired equilibrium is reestablished. And so goes the cycle of life, eh? We are constantly striving to regain our balance after something rocks our world. So stress is a consistent part of life, and not always bad. Stress can add excitement to life. Gets the blood pumping and the juices flowing. But, in the context of caregiving, chronic stress can have detrimental consequences. In order to mitigate the ripples and waves in the pond, we need to identify and control the sources of stress (pebbles and rocks). We can only rock and roll for so long before becoming seasick.

Stress

A person's response to a destabilizing force. Illness and the complications associated with advanced age are certainly destabilizing forces. Get ready for a few waves in your pond!

Definition

Boomers, we have lived long enough to know how we typically manifest stress. I typically get migraines when I'm stressed out. That is my Red Flag Warning that I'm ignoring the waves in my pond. Now, I'm the first one to admit that there are times when I ignore the warning. I choose to keep doing what I'm doing for whatever reason. And when I do that, I pay the price. I have a raging migraine for weeks. The point being, we make choices and live with the consequences. In the context of caregiving, there are times when we get so consumed by the task at hand that we fail to see the warning signs. We are so focused on the well-being of our loved one that we neglect to "see" our own needs. We can usually handle this for short periods of time without life-altering consequences. However, the chronic stress of long-term caregiving poses a significant risk. Caregiving can rub you raw. Have some healing balm handy.

The Risks of Caregiving

Why should you be interested in the topic of caregiving stress? What difference does it make to you, whether caregiver or care receiver? Let me highlight the importance of stress management and mitigation by articulating what you risk losing if ignorant of this important issue. Stress that is unrecognized, untreated, and uncontrolled poses a huge risk to you and your family. Both caregivers and care receivers risk losing the sense of physical, emotional, spiritual, psychosocial, and financial well-being. Quality of life is compromised to the extreme. The greatest risk in the primary caregiver-care receiver scenario is that the primary caregiver has a serious health care crisis or predeceases the care receiver due to unmitigated stress. When that happens (and it does), a caregiving crisis ensues that escalates the stress level for all involved. Not pretty. Do I have your attention?

I invite you to carefully consider all aspects of your current or future caregiving situation. Identify the stressors. Recognize the risks of chronic stress. Then sit back and weigh your options. It's just like investing in the stock market. You research the various investment options. You understand the risks and the rewards. You establish your investment goals. Then you do a gut check. How much risk are you willing to assume? Once determined, you can make well-informed decisions. Even though there are no guarantees, you're working to limit your risks while maximizing the rewards. The same is true for caregiving. Ask yourself these questions. Is this an investment I choose to make? Or is this an investment I have to make (caregiver by default)? Is this a short-term or long-term investment? Based on your answers, invest yourself wisely into the process of caregiving. Do your research. Identify the risks and rewards. And then determine how much risk you're willing to tolerate. Just like the stock market, caregiving is inherently risky. Have realistic expectations. The challenge, and the opportunity, is risk management.

Care Receiver—Possible Stressors

The care receiver is a critical character in the caregiving scenario. Shocking but true! All the practical aspects of the person come to bear on the complexities of care—who, what, when, where, why, how, and for how long. But there are other factors to consider. Will the care receiver willingly accept help from others or stubbornly refuse? Is the care receiver a pleasant or ornery individual? Is there a strong, emotional bond between caregiver and care receiver? Does the family *want* to care for this person? Important questions to consider as you ponder the future caregiving needs of your aging family members (and yourself). What other attributes of the care receiver impact the stress of caregiving? Let's consider the following items.

Get Real

Several years ago, I presented a program on caregiving to families confronted by the challenges of dementia. At one point in the program, I acknowledged that caregiving can be incredibly difficult at times. However, there are also blessings to be derived from the experience as well. At this point, one of the caregivers in the room raised her hand to get my attention. She asked if she could offer a different perspective of caregiving. Her courageous, raw insights of caregiving resonated with all in the room.

She served as the primary caregiver for her mother who was diagnosed with a rare form of dementia five years ago. Since the diagnosis, life had become an endless series of frightening changes. Her mother was no longer the person she had known and loved for fifty years. Now there were days she didn't even like her mother. Every day, there was something else her mother couldn't do or couldn't remember. She concluded by saying, "Right now, caregiving is just hard. There are no blessings. There is no joy. And that's just the way it is for now. Perhaps ten years from now, I'll be able to look back and discover something of value. But today, I am too close to see the blessings. My focus is on getting through the next hour without falling apart." With that, she sat back and awaited my response.

I had no response. Instead, I was humbled by her realistic, honest assessment of the situation. Having been in the trenches with my own mother, I knew what she meant. When you're knee-deep in the muck of caregiving, your focus is on the next step. The blessings of the journey, if any, are saved for another day. This woman taught me, in no uncertain terms, that to idealize the journey of caregiving is to diminish the price paid by caregivers and care receivers alike. To fast forward to the blessings and the rewards of caregiving is to disregard the current risks. I am forever grateful for having met this woman. I now resist the temptation to sanitize caregiving. Honesty is the best policy, right? So know going in, you'll probably need your hip waders and a shovel. It can get pretty nasty in the trenches. Forewarned is forearmed!

Role in the Family/Family History

In **Chapter 4**, we discussed the wonderful world of families. We explored how the challenges posed by aging and illness serve to destabilize the entire family system. One of the determining factors as to the extent and duration of disruption is the role of the care receiver. Has this person historically been the decision maker in the family? Communicator? Spiritual leader? Will these roles be reassigned to other family members? And if so, for how long? Role changes are tremendously stressful for all involved, whether temporary or permanent.

Also, for families with histories of abuse or addiction, the stress can be magnified when a caregiving issue arises. Family secrets bubble to the surface and old wounds are exposed. Imagine a daughter, who was sexually abused by her father, being asked to serve as her father's caregiver. What if no one in the family is aware of the past abuse? Will the family accept the daughter's refusal to care for her father or instead push her to help? I mention this possible scenario to highlight an important facet of caregiving— it is complicated. Even in your own family, you don't know everything about everyone! There are stories and family history driving many of the choices made regarding caregiving. So instead of judging someone's ability or inability to care, perhaps we are better served to honor their boundaries and honest response.

Relationship to Caregiver

From my experience, the nature of the relationship between the care receiver and the caregiver(s) is a significant factor in the level of stress experienced by both. When there is an attitude of mutual respect, mutual affection, and mutual concern, the level of stress is tolerable. When absent, stress can become unbearable and relationships irreparably harmed.

Financial Resources

Health care expenses are a major source of stress for most families. There is a pervasive fear of outliving our financial resources and then becoming dependent on our families or governmental programs such as Medicaid. The reality is that most people in our country are one major illness away from bankruptcy! So the financial resources of the care receiver are vitally

Alone for Good Reason

Mrs. Gordon was an incredibly bitter, angry woman. And for good reason, according to her. She was alone in life. Although she had children and siblings, she hadn't spoken to them in years. They abandoned her! She played the role of victim quite well. When I met her, she was in her mideighties with a variety of chronic conditions. She resided in an assisted living community that provided excellent care. As her chaplain, I listened to many a story about the failings of her family. If that wasn't enough venom for the day, she launched into stories about the nursing staff at the facility. Although I lamented the fact that this woman was alone at the end of her life, I also recognized her role in that reality. We do truly reap what we sow in this life. A reminder to plant good seeds along the way!

Uninspired

important when developing a plan of care. If funds are limited, the financial stress of caregiving radiates throughout the family system.

Friends and Colleagues

As discussed in **Chapter 2**, the family unit has changed dramatically over the past fifty years. Our families are typically smaller and scattered across the globe. Hence, most of us don't have an abundance of family members waiting in the wings to come to our aid when needed. Consequently, when a caregiving issue arises, care receivers may rely on friends and colleagues for a significant amount of care. Due to the geographic dispersal of families, friends often serve as the eyes, ears, and hands for long-distance caregivers. You know well the adage that you can't have too many friends, right? Truer words were never spoken when it comes to caregiving! You will need more help than you ever imagined!

Attitude

When working as a hospice chaplain, I scheduled my appointments in a very specific way. I saved my favorite families for the last visit of the day. I did this for a couple of reasons. First, I could extend the visit without worry about subsequent appointments. Second, by the end of the day, I needed and wanted to be around positive, life-giving people. I was blessed to share many an afternoon with gracious, kind, loving, and compassionate people. People who welcomed me into their homes and into their lives. The people who drew me in were those who chose to embrace life. They were not embittered by life, victims of circumstances. Rather, they courageously confronted the reality of their mortality and taught me what it meant to be fully present to the moment. The attitude of care receivers can either draw people in or send them running for the hills! So, my friends, choose wisely. Attitude *is* everything!

Caregiving Situation—Possible Stressors

The level of stress experienced by caregivers and receivers is highly influenced by the specifics of care. Are you contemplating a short-term recovery from hip surgery? Or is your family confronted by the long and problematic journey of dementia? Pebble or rock in the pond? Also, depending on the relationship between caregiver and care receiver, certain types of intimate care may cause distress. So it is important to recognize potential sources of stress related to the specifics of care. Once identified, seek alternatives to reduce the level of stress and thus enhance the quality of life for the caregiver and care receiver. Remember, proactive beats reactive every time. So anticipate the potential stressors of caregiving and seek effective alternatives. Some things to consider:

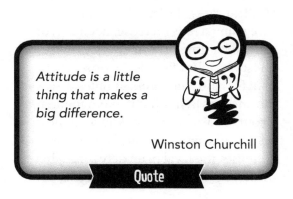

Attitude is a little thing that makes a big difference.

Winston Churchill

Quote

Diagnosis/Medical Concern

What is the diagnosis or medical concern? Is the condition a physical, cognitive, or mental health issue? The diagnosis obviously has direct implications on the type of care, duration of care, and prognosis. As noted previously, knowledge of the disease process allows families to proactively plan for future caregiving needs. Families capable of anticipating needs experience significantly less stress than those reacting to changing conditions. Additionally, proactive or not, it is well documented that dementia care is significantly more stressful than other types of care due to the intensity and duration of care. Primary caregivers of persons with dementia might want to consider sharing the responsibility of care with other family members and professional caregivers.

Prognosis

Is the diagnosis a curable, chronic, or terminal illness? The nature of the illness relates to the anticipated duration of caregiving as well as the expected outcome. When dealing with a chronic or terminal condition, families are doing much more than meeting the basic, daily needs of the care receiver. Everyone involved is preparing for the ultimate change—death. That is a daunting, emotional task indeed. As we know, caregiving journeys that entail significant or continuous change prove to be the most stressful. The family is in a constant state of flux. Families dealing with chronic, progressive, and terminal illness can't get too comfortable. Change is a'coming!

Change Fatigue

One of the more challenging aspects of chronic and progressive illness is incessant change. With every change in the physical or cognitive status of the care receiver, the precarious equilibrium of the family is disrupted. The transition time after the change is a time of rebalancing, relearning, and reknowing. Over time, people become weary of change and the constant need to readjust. This is referred to as *change fatigue* and can cause people to become even more resistant to change. This is when realistic expectations and knowledge of the disease process are critically important. Change *is* to be expected. Change *is* the norm.

Perspiration

Level/Type of Care Needed

Will the care receiver require 24/7 care? Medical care? Nonmedical care? Will the caregiving needs increase, decrease, or cease over time? The answers to these questions allow families to proactively plan for care. Too often, families discover the answers in midflight, often mandating a course correction. Not knowing the details of what, how, and for how long increases the level of anxiety throughout the family. As always, knowledge is power.

Duration of Care

Based on the diagnosis and prognosis, will the caregiving journey be a short- or long-term proposition? Your plan of care is contingent on the level and duration of care. In **Part 4**, we'll explore the option of sharing the responsibilities of care with a caring community. This is one way to reduce the stress of a long-term caregiving journey.

Caregiver(s)—Possible Stressors

Thus far, we've discussed how the care receiver and the specifics of care can either increase or decrease the level of stress. Now we need to consider how the caregiver(s) can impact the overall experience of caregiving. For the purposes of our discussion, I'll assume there is a primary caregiver. Let's consider the various characteristics that either serve to increase or decrease the stress of caregiving.

Relationship/Gender

Women and men share the duties of caregiving, currently estimated at a 60/40 split. Both male and female caregivers can provide exceptional care. However, there may be situations in which the gender of the caregiver increases the stress for those involved. For example, a daughter bathing a father. A son caring for a mother who is incontinent. In situations like this, it's important to recognize your boundaries. It's okay to state that you're uncomfortable doing certain things. You can then determine how best to proceed.

Age

Although the average age of caregivers in the United States is 48, people of all ages provide care for a loved one. Extreme age, very young or very old, can become a significant stressor. Children do not have the maturity or life experiences to deal well with all the issues associated with illness and aging. The elderly often have their own health concerns to contend with while caring for another. Either situation creates additional stress for those involved.

Health Status—Abilities and Disabilities

Caregiving is a challenging endeavor made only more difficult if the caregiver has health concerns or is at a physical disadvantage. Is the caregiver able (physically and/or cognitively) to administer the care required? Women caring for men often find transfers physically difficult if not impossible. Once again, it is important to recognize our limitations and plan accordingly.

Experience

Whether applying for a job or serving as a caregiver, experience is important. Your past experience serves to prepare you for current and future challenges. Are you a novice at caregiving and therefore apprehensive and anxious? Or are you a seasoned veteran of past caregiving journeys, confident you can meet any challenge? Confidence in your abilities, whether novice or veteran, serves to reduce your overall level of stress.

Pure Genius!

He Stays!

Michael was in a heated debate with the nurse when he heard the soft, but firm, voice of his mother. He knew that voice well after sixty years. His mother was taking control even as she lay in her hospital bed. No surprise to Michael! A few moments before, the nurse entered the room to examine his mother and had requested Michael leave the room. Since Michael was the primary caregiver for his mother, he refused to leave. He wanted to witness the exam and be privy to the conversation. The nurse obviously thought it was inappropriate for "the son" to be in the room during the exam.

His mother proceeded to tell the nurse that her son had been instrumental in her care for over five years. In fact, Michael had overseen all aspects of her care, ensuring everything was done correctly. Michael routinely emptied her catheter. He administered drugs. When needed, he cleaned and dressed wounds. He came by daily to rub lotion on her feet and back. And he even bathed her when the CNA called in sick a few weeks ago. So if she had an issue with her son being in the room, the nurse had two choices. She could get over her bias against male caregivers and get on with the exam or she could leave and send in another nurse. *He stays!*

The rest of the story? Michael stayed. The nurse completed the exam. Recommendations were discussed. A care receiver and caregiver were honored. A nurse broadened her understanding and appreciation of caregivers. And perhaps that nurse will think twice before asking family members to leave the room. A better approach? Ask the care receiver what is preferred. All good things.

Training

Knowledge instills confidence in caregivers. Thus, appropriate training of caregivers serves to reduce stress. As a caregiver, if you feel ill equipped or incapable of providing the needed care, *ask* for the needed assistance and instruction.

Attitude

The attitude of the caregiver is equally as important as the attitude of the care receiver. Your attitude influences the process. Granted, due to the nature of caregiving, some days will be better than others. But, overall, how do you approach the journey? How do you "feel" as a caregiver?

Employment/Financial Resources

Serving as a caregiver is a costly proposition. It is known that 60 percent of caregivers work full time. If called to care, how is your job impacted by the additional responsibilities of caregiving?

- Increased absenteeism
- Diminished productivity
- Extended leave
- Reluctance to assume heavier workload
- Resistance to transfers and promotions
- Resignation (leave the workforce)

MetLife conducted a study in 2011 to determine the financial costs for men and women (aged fifty and older) leaving the workforce to care for a loved one. The aggregate costs included lost wages, reduction in pension, and adjustments to social security benefits. The average

My Aching Back

A very common complaint of caregivers is back pain. This is true for personal as well as professional caregivers. When transferring care receivers, caregivers should employ appropriate lifting techniques and equipment to ensure the safety of the caregiver and care receiver. This is not a trial-and-error type of training! Proactively seek the needed training to avoid serious injury.

Observation

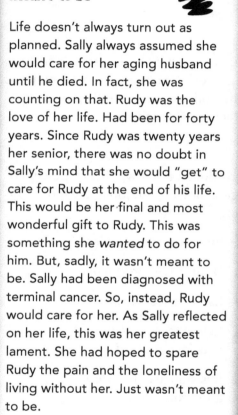

Wasn't Meant to Be

Life doesn't always turn out as planned. Sally always assumed she would care for her aging husband until he died. In fact, she was counting on that. Rudy was the love of her life. Had been for forty years. Since Rudy was twenty years her senior, there was no doubt in Sally's mind that she would "get" to care for Rudy at the end of his life. This would be her final and most wonderful gift to Rudy. This was something she *wanted* to do for him. But, sadly, it wasn't meant to be. Sally had been diagnosed with terminal cancer. So, instead, Rudy would care for her. As Sally reflected on her life, this was her greatest lament. She had hoped to spare Rudy the pain and the loneliness of living without her. Just wasn't meant to be.

> **Example**

aggregate costs totaled $304,000 per person. Obviously, this directly impacts the ability of the caregiver to meet current and future personal financial obligations. Stress rises! Caregiving is hard enough physically and emotionally. The addition of financial stress multiples the problems.

Family Situation

Caregiver is not your only role in life, right? You have other roles and responsibilities within your family. How will those be affected by your role as caregiver? Who or what gets shortchanged as you reallocate time and energy? Are you married or in relationship? Do you have children? Are the other people in your life supportive of your role as caregiver? If not, the stress and strain on your personal relationships will enhance the stress of the caregiving journey. Your role as caregiver impacts everyone you know and love. Don't ignore the ripples on your pond! Many a family has been pulled asunder by the challenges of caregiving. Work collaboratively to support one another throughout the journey.

Local or Long Distance

In **Chapter 6**, we talked extensively about the issue of long-distance caregiving. The geographic separation between caregiver and care receiver increases the financial stress (travel expenses), physical stress (traveling), and emotional stress (guilt for not being there). In contrast, local caregivers experience the stress of constant care. Resentment arises if the local caregivers feel unsupported and unappreciated by long-distance family members. Local caregivers often assume the role by default, feeling as if they have no choice in the matter. Whether a local or long-distance caregiver, there is more than enough stress to go around.

Cultural and Family Norms and Expectations

Is there an expectation within your family as to who will serve as a caregiver? Is it shameful to ask nonfamily members to assist with care? This may be part of your family legacy. Or perhaps this shame is a cultural norm. In

Example

Drained Dry

Eileen looked at her reflection in the mirror. What she saw was frightening. She had aged so much over the past five years. It had been difficult on so many levels. Caring for her aging parents as the only child, she carried the load. Her responsibility. Her honor. A few years ago, she moved in with her parents to alleviate the stress of travel. She had grown weary of the transcontinental flights. Her employer had grown equally weary of her frequent absences. At the time, she felt confident she could get back into the workforce after her parents died. She was a top producer and highly sought after by other Fortune 500 companies. Additionally, she was assured of a sizable inheritance. The plan seemed reasonable.

Today, she realized the tragic flaws in her logic. She failed to comprehend the level, intensity, duration, and cost of care her parents ultimately required. Not only did her parents drain their financial reservoirs, but Eileen's financial resources were depleted as well. She wasn't angry with her parents. They were dear souls. Instead, she was jealous of them. They didn't have to deal with her financial devastation. They didn't have to start over. But she did. How does a sixty-two-year-old unemployed woman reenter the workforce? Eileen was about to find out. One step at a time. She might be financially drained, but she was determined to persevere. That is the one thing she did inherit from her parents—a steely will and the determination to thrive. Attributes she would need in the days ahead.

cases where family or cultural norms prohibit others from helping, the responsibility of care resides on the shoulders of family members only. Depending on the circumstances, families may opt to modify historical norms in order to meet the current needs.

Availability of Family Caregivers

If you serve as a primary caregiver, you will probably need or want backup. Are there other members of your family willing to serve as caregivers? Sharing the responsibility of care with family, friends, and/or professional services is one of the best ways to reduce the stress of caregiving. Something to consider.

Geographic Location—Possible Stressors

In **Chapter 10**, we discussed the implications of geographic location on caregiving. Henry and Carmen's choice to live in a small, coastal village served them well until Carmen suffered a stroke. Due to limited caregiving resources, they were forced to relocate. Henry and Carmen took a risk. They risked living in a place they loved that ultimately could not accommodate acute health care needs. But if you asked Henry and Carmen, it might have been worth the risk for the time they enjoyed on the coast. It's all about balancing the risks and rewards.

Expressions of Stress—Red Flag Warnings

To this point, we've identified the various factors that serve to intensify the level of stress for caregivers and care receivers. We've also acknowledged that unrecognized, uncontrolled, and unmitigated stress threatens to compromise the well-being of all involved. Therefore, recognizing the warning signs in ourselves and others is the first step in addressing our stress. How do you typically respond to stress? What emotions are triggered by stress? What behaviors reflect an inability to manage stress? These are the signs that serve as the Red Flag Warnings, the indicators that stress is on the rise. We are wise to heed these warnings and subsequently address our stress.

Physical signs:

- Compromised immune system
- Gastrointestinal issues
- Increased frequency of health issues
- Cardiac issues
- Aches and pains

Cognitive signs:

- Memory impairment
- Fearfulness
- Increased anxiety
- Pessimism

Emotional signs:

- Anger
- Moodiness
- Frustration
- Feeling overwhelmed
- Impatience
- Helplessness
- Irritability
- Grief
- Depression

Behavioral signs:

- Abusive behaviors (physical and emotional)
- Drug and alcohol abuse
- Lack of personal hygiene
- Changes in sleep habits
- Changes in eating habits
- Isolation and social withdrawal
- Nervous habits
- Overly controlling of people and situations

I Did It My Way!

I have already admitted that I am somewhat of a control queen. I will also admit that when stressed, I become even more controlling. This is not an uncommon reaction to stress. It actually makes a lot of sense when confronted by the challenges of illness and aging. When we can't control the progression of an illness, we *can* control the minutia in life. When we can't stop age from progressing, we *can* attempt to control the people in our lives. We control what we can! It may seem silly in hindsight. But at the time, it makes all the sense in the world. And it means the world to us! Let me give you an example.

When I was nineteen, I was preparing the house for my mom's homecoming. She had been in the hospital for over a week following extensive surgery. I was an emotional wreck. Earlier in the week, I learned she had less than two years to live. And that was questionable, according to the oncologist. I didn't know how to deal with that reality, so I focused on what I could control. I cleaned the house from top to bottom. I mowed the yard. I mopped the floors. I cooked an incredible meal. And I hung the wash on the line to dry. My mom needed fresh, clean linens for her homecoming. I could control that. That I could do.

As I was dashing about, the doorbell rang. A dear friend of my mom's stopped by to help me. Understand, I needed no help. I had everything under control! This dear woman sensed my resistance and did her best not to ruffle my feathers. Seeing the sheets on the line, she offered to make my mom's bed. While she did that, I busied myself in the kitchen putting the finishing touches on dinner. However, I just couldn't resist overseeing the bed-making process. As I entered my parent's bedroom, I witnessed the top sheet being place "print down" on the bed. What? That is *not* how you make a bed! The top sheet is placed "print up" on the bed. Everyone knows that. My mom's friend assured me that up or down, the sheet served the same purpose. Realizing I was not going to win the argument, I left the room with dramatic flair. Shortly thereafter, the woman said goodbye and wished us a lovely reunion.

I am sure you can guess the end of this story. The minute the front door closed, I dashed back to the bedroom, ripped off the sheets, and made the bed the *right* way. I couldn't control my mom's cancer. I couldn't save her from a certain death. But, I could control how my mom's bed was made. In that moment, it mattered. I did it my way. And I would do it again!

At this point, you are probably wondering who in their right mind would *ever* consider being a caregiver. Why take the risk? Well, I hope you know by now that I am a champion for caregiving. I think there is no higher calling in this life than to companion another person in the caregiving journey. But to serve well, we must engage caregiving with our eyes wide open. We must see the blessings as well as the pitfalls. Having a heightened awareness of the risks posed by elevated levels of stress enables caregivers to recognize the warning signs of stress gone wild. Once seen, we can then be intentional about addressing our stress. In **Chapter 15**, we'll explore some ideas on how to mitigate stress. However, before that, I want to discuss a specific type of stress that family and professional caregivers are at risk of experiencing: compassion fatigue. Keep reading. I promise it won't be too stressful!

To Summarize...

- Caregiving is a stressful proposition for all involved, caregiver and care receiver. It's not enough to merely acknowledge that the journey is stressful. We need to realize the risk involved if we choose to ignore the implications of chronic stress. Knowing what we have to lose should be motivation enough to address our stress.

- Stress is the response to a destabilizing force in life. When a pebble falls into your peaceful pond, the ripples and waves rock your world. Your challenge is to regain a sense of equilibrium and carry on. How you choose to cope and adapt to the destabilizing force informs your overall experience.

- Stress is a part of life. It's a given. So, in the context of caregiving, we need to identify the various sources of stress. By knowing the source of our stress, we can hopefully manage the number of pebbles falling into the pond and the frequency at which they fall.

- No matter how knowledgeable and how proactive we are, we will experience some level of caregiving stress. Hence, we need to be aware of the signs that stress is rising to critical levels. By knowing the physical, emotional, cognitive, and behavioral manifestations of stress, we can recognize the signs of stress gone wild and choose to address our stress.

Chapter 14

Compassion Fatigue

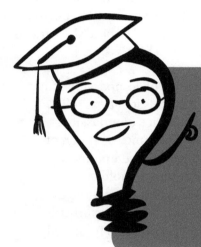

In This Chapter...

- What is compassion fatigue?
- How do you recognize compassion fatigue?
- Why are boundaries important?
- What can be done to alleviate compassion fatigue?

Compassion fatigue may be an unfamiliar term. However, I can guarantee that you have experienced this particular type of stress as a caregiver. Witnessing the journey of the aged and the ill profoundly affects us. As compassionate beings, we long to help those in need. However, despite our best intentions, there are situations we can't fix. Suffering we can't relieve. Our inability to resolve the suffering often results in compassion fatigue. Compassion fatigue ultimately reduces our capacity to care, a serious concern for caregivers!

As with all types of stress, recognition is the first order of business. How do we recognize compassion fatigue? Well, in all honesty, the Red Flag Warnings of chronic stress noted in **Chapter 13** are consistent for all types of stress.

Once stress is recognized, the challenge is then to determine the source and subsequent type of stress. Compassion fatigue is rooted in our overidentification with and/or overexposure to the suffering of others. In the case of family caregivers, the source of stress is then fairly obvious—witnessing the suffering of an aged or ill family member. Within the context of compassion fatigue, we can then begin to understand the "whys" behind the various manifestations of stress.

Compassion Fatigue

Also referred to as secondary traumatic stress and vicarious trauma, compassion fatigue is a condition resulting from the overexposure to and/or overidentification with the suffering of others (people and animals). Compassion fatigue ultimately reduces our capacity to care.

Definition

Exposing the roots of compassion fatigue reveals opportunities for stress relief. Caregivers experience compassion fatigue when we assume too much of the emotional load and responsibility for the journey. Our empathy goes into overdrive. We must then be mindful of what is ours to hold and what is not. Therefore, well-established and maintained boundaries serve us well. We also experience compassion fatigue as a result of overexposure to the suffering of others. Thus, it is important for caregivers to frequently disconnect from the role of caregiver.

Compassion Fatigue

Compassion fatigue is a hot topic within the ranks of professional caregivers. However, *all* caregivers are at risk of experiencing compassion fatigue. *Compassion fatigue* is experienced as a result of overexposure to and/or overidentification with the suffering of others (people and animals). By witnessing the suffering of others, we are vicariously traumatized. Consequently, compassion fatigue is often referred to as secondary traumatic stress. As caregivers, we have experienced, we are experiencing, or we will experience compassion fatigue. 'Tis the nature of the journey. We'll witness too much. Take on too much. Feel too much. Because we care too much. We do this because we are compassionate, empathetic beings. Ultimately, by raising our awareness to this concern, we'll be better able to recognize the signs of compassion fatigue in ourselves and others. Later in this chapter, we'll discuss effective ways to address this type of stress.

Compassion

The concept of compassion is elemental to the understanding of compassion fatigue. *Compassion* literally means to bear or to suffer with. As compassionate people, we are moved emotionally by the suffering of others. Every day, we experience countless, compassionate responses to the things going on in the world. Images of tragic events on the Internet. A homeless person standing on the corner with a cardboard sign. An abandoned puppy seeking shelter. A care receiver moaning in pain before the morphine takes effect. Because we are compassionate, we *feel* a bit of the pain we witness.

Compassion entails more than an emotional reaction. It is also a relational response. So, when emotionally moved by the suffering of others, we are motivated to *do* something to alleviate the suffering. Images on the Internet prompt a donation to a relief fund. A homeless person receives money or a bottle of water. A frightened puppy finds a forever family. A care receiver knows the blessing of a courageous companion. As witnesses to suffering, our compassion prompts us to *do* something.

Our desire to alleviate suffering exposes us to the possibility of compassion fatigue. We witness a disturbing situation, and we want to *fix* it. But some situations are not fixable. Some situations are beyond our control. When caring for people we love, this is a particularly harsh reality to accept. If we are unwilling or unable to acknowledge our limitations, the risk of compassion fatigue becomes the reality.

Empathy

Empathy is the capacity to relate to another's situation and emotions. Empathy serves all those in the helping professions. To serve well, we must be able to relate to the other person. However, a strength overplayed becomes a weakness. Such is the case with empathy and suffering. If we overidentify with the suffering of others, empathy triggers compassion fatigue.

Basically, empathy serves as an accelerant for compassion, like throwing gasoline on a fire. The burning desire to "fix" a situation burns white hot when we understand the situation from the inside out. Empathy is our visceral response. We have been there, done that. We know what the other person feels, because we have felt the same thing! The danger arises when empathy blurs the line between caregiver and care receiver. When boundaries blur, it is hard to know what is ours to bear and what is not. In our overzealous desire to help, we compromise our effectiveness and our well-being. Thus, boundaries are of preeminent importance when it comes to compassion fatigue. If we cross the line, even with the best of intentions, our risk of experiencing compassion fatigue escalates exponentially.

Who Is at Risk?

No one is immune to compassion fatigue. But there are certain professions and roles that are at greater risk of experiencing compassion fatigue than others. Caregivers, personal and professional, are obviously at high risk for vicarious trauma. So, if you are skimming this chapter thinking I am not speaking to you, wake up! This is a concern for everyone. Even you! I don't care how many times you've been a caregiver. I don't care if you have six academic degrees and a string of letters after your name. I don't care how much you know about caregiving. When exposed to enough suffering and loss for an extended period of time, we are all at risk of experiencing compassion fatigue. So pay attention!

There is another reason to become knowledgeable about compassion

I Couldn't *Fix* It

After forty-eight hours of my mom's relentless nausea, diarrhea, and vomiting caused by radical chemotherapy, I sat on the bathroom floor cradling her head in my lap. We were physically exhausted, emotionally ravaged, and spiritually numb. As I stroked her head, strands of her hair fell out and onto my bathrobe. Words today cannot begin to capture the horror, the betrayal, the anger, and the rage I felt. The past four months had been brutal. Biopsies. Surgery. Consultations. Chemotherapy. Suffering. I looked at my mom, wondering how much more she could take. She had been through hell and back. In that moment, I would have given my life to change her reality. But even at nineteen, I knew that wasn't possible. I couldn't *fix* it. That realization proved to be my own version of hell for the next five years.

Example

I Know How You Feel

When Helen introduced me to her daughter, Emily, alarm bells went off in my head. I felt as if I'd been transported back in time. As I chatted briefly with Emily, I saw myself in her. Emily was eighteen. She obviously adored her mother. And she served as her mother's caregiver since the diagnosis of metastatic breast cancer. In order to "hear" their story, I had to mute the old tapes playing in my head. I had to keep reminding myself that this was not me. Helen was not my mom. This was not *my* story. But the situation was so similar. My heart broke for them. I kept thinking, "I know how you feel." But did I? Perhaps, to a certain extent. I could empathize with Emily because I had been a caregiver for my own mother. But I had to allow Emily to be Emily. She didn't need to carry the burden of my story. Nor did I need to carry the burden of hers.

Example

fatigue. We can serve as mirrors for our family members, friends, and colleagues. Sometimes it is much easier to "see" compassion fatigue in another person than in ourselves. Always true, right? I recognize the signs in others much more readily than in myself. This is important. The sooner we recognize the signs, the sooner we can work to mitigate the stress. So, as a family, watch for the signs of compassion fatigue in each other. Sometimes, self-care is a collaborative process.

If no one is immune to compassion fatigue, what about care *receivers*? Well, I think we need to consider this question carefully. What leads to compassion fatigue? Overidentification with and/or overexposure to the suffering of another. Now, let's consider the caregiving situation from the perspective of the care *receiver*. For example, what does a gentleman with advanced Parkinson's disease witness every day? Perhaps he sees his wife struggling to care for him, the house, the bills, and a job. Maybe he sees the sadness in the eyes of his children when he can no longer walk. On occasion, he senses the fear of his family as his condition worsens. Is the gentleman a witness to tremendous suffering? Is this a chronic type of stress? Could he possibly overidentify with the suffering of his family? *Yes*! Absolutely! Yes ma'am! Amen!

Please, recognize that care *receivers* are at high risk of compassion fatigue as well. Yes, the perspective is quite different. But the signs of compassion fatigue are the same. Pay attention to the Red Flag Warnings.

Red Flag Warnings of Compassion Fatigue

In **Chapter 13**, I listed the various signs of stress: physical, emotional, cognitive, and behavioral. The signs for compassion fatigue are quite similar to those previously listed. However, it is important to understand why certain signs of stress are particularly common with compassion fatigue. Knowing the sources of compassion fatigue, you will no doubt discern the relationship between the causes of compassion fatigue and the signs of stress. But just in case you don't, I'll provide some additional food for thought. In all instances, pay attention to deviations from the norm in yourself and your family. The deviations serve as your Red Flag Warnings. The signs of compassion fatigue include:

> ## Remember Care Receivers
>
> Discussions of compassion fatigue usually focus on the caregiver's experience. It's important to realize that care receivers experience compassion fatigue as well.
>
> **IMPORTANT!**

- Overwhelmed and barely hanging on. When companioning someone with long-term caregiving needs, we witness a tremendous amount of change, loss, and suffering. We often feel that just one more thing will push us over the edge. So we hang on for dear life. The "waiting for the other shoe to drop" kind of existence generates tremendous anxiety within a family.

- Irritated, anxious, and fearful. Overexposure to stress tends to make us feel vulnerable and at risk. Additionally, we become irritated that there is little we can do to change the situation. We can't *fix* it. This can create tremendous tension within a family as caregivers become impatient and short tempered.

- Angry. Anger is an interesting emotion, one most people don't handle well. Anger is neither good nor bad. It is how we express anger that determines the merits of the emotion. Additionally, there is always another emotion beneath the anger that drives our rage. We are angry *because* we feel out of control, at risk, frustrated, ineffective,

Look Beyond the Anger

Anger is a problematic emotion for most people. We don't know how to deal well with anger. However, knowing that anger is the outward manifestation of another emotion is helpful. Then, instead of reacting to the anger, we can choose to look beyond the rage to discover the underlying issue: fear, frustration, loss of control, grief, and sadness.

Observation

powerless, incapable, helpless, or afraid. Thus, compassion fatigue naturally generates feelings of anger because of our impotence to change the situation. Instead of ignoring anger, I find it to be an incredibly helpful signal. It is the fire alarm that alerts me to the fact that there is something else going on, something deeper that I need to examine. If you can work through the anger to uncover the reason for the anger, then you can make some progress on alleviating your stress.

- **Overly emotional.** Have you ever had an occasion when an insignificant blip on your radar screen caused a massive meltdown? And, no, I'm not talking about menopause! Stay focused. We're talking about compassion fatigue. Witnessing the suffering of others takes a toll on caregivers—physically, emotionally, and spiritually. So an occasional meltdown is not out of the question. In fact, moving the energy and emotions around is often quite therapeutic. Sometimes we just need to let 'er rip!

- **Depressed.** Depression is a significant risk for all caregivers. This is more than feeling occasionally blue or down. I am referring to clinical depression, which mandates professional help and possibly medications. Compassion fatigue can result in depression when a caregiver feels that all efforts to alleviate suffering are futile. All is lost. And thus the caregiver despairs.

- **Isolated and withdrawn.** Caregiving, in general, can lead to isolation and withdrawal due to lack of time and energy. With compassion fatigue, this sign can be indicative of many things: apathy, fear, despair, fatigue, and anxiety. The behavior merely indicates that something is going on. We must then explore the underlying cause for the isolation and withdrawal.

Frequent medical issues. Compassion fatigue is a specific type of chronic stress. And as we know, chronic stress compromises the immune system. Caregivers are thus at increased risk of experiencing their own health care crisis in the midst of the caregiving journey. If you are a frequent visitor to your primary care doctor or emergency clinic, pay attention. This could be a precursor to a medical emergency.

Excessive behaviors. Those suffering from compassion fatigue often obsess on the source of the suffering, consumed by thoughts and emotions. In order to get away from the stress, we need a distraction. We distract ourselves with food, gambling, sex, exercise, alcohol, drugs, and work. Some of these excesses become life-threatening and relationship-breaking addictions.

Changes in sleep habits. Again, we are looking at deviations from normal behaviors. You are sleeping either too much or too little as a result of compassion fatigue. You may walk the floors due to an increased level of anxiety. Or you can't get out of bed due to apathy, fatigue, and despair. Either extreme will usually be recognized first by your family. Changes in sleep habits disrupt the normal family rhythms.

Blaming others. Blaming others is a very common sign of compassion fatigue. Why? Well, consider this. You are doing everything you can to alleviate the suffering of your loved one. Despite your efforts, the situation remains the same. You can't fix it. So you need someone or something to blame for this failure. You blame the health care providers. You blame family members who aren't working as hard as you. You blame the care receiver for not trying hard enough. And on

Out of Sight, Out of Mind

It is far too easy for caregivers to isolate unnoticed. This is particularly true for long-term caregivers. It's not that family, friends, and colleagues don't care. People just get busy living their own lives. So I invite you to do an occasional pulse check on the caregivers in your life. A phone call, text, or email is a gift, indeed, for an isolated caregiver.

Inspiration

and on. Obviously, this blame game can destroy relationships and generate additional stress in families and organizations (professional caregivers). So, if you find yourself wagging a finger at someone, see the bigger point! You are probably frustrated that you cannot alleviate the suffering of a loved one. You can't change the reality of the situation. You can't *fix* it. No one is to blame.

The Beauty of Boundaries

Have you ever found yourself saying, "I know *exactly* how you feel. That happened to me." Sure you have. We all have. This is an empathic response. I recognize how you feel, because I've felt similarly. We stand on common ground, but not the exact same piece of ground. So I can relate to you, but I'm *not* you! This distinction is vitally important for caregivers, personal and professional. If I am mindful of the boundary between you and me, I can distinguish my journey from yours. I may have traveled a similar road in times past, but I can't save you from all the twists and turns, the potholes, and the suffering. Interjecting myself into *your* story changes the narrative and clutters the path. Your suffering is not mine to bear. No matter how desperately I want to help you. There are times when I can only witness your suffering. I cannot change your reality, but I can companion you. One step at a time.

Boundaries are the blessed friends of caregivers. Well-established, maintained boundaries keep us literally "between the lines." Boundaries delineate our interactions with others. What is appropriate. What is not. What is beneficial. What is not. In the context of compassion fatigue, boundaries keep our empathy in check. Each time we bump into a boundary, we are reminded of where we reside. The particular piece of ground on which we stand. As long as we stay grounded, we can serve well.

I'm Walking the Floor Over You

If you find yourself reciting infomercials or wearing a path in the carpet because you can't sleep, it's time to take stock of your situation. What's going on? Although it's a catchy tune, "walking the floor over you" is no way to dance through life.

Example

Diagnosis Compassion Fatigue— What Now?

After reading this chapter, have you self-diagnosed compassion fatigue? Maybe you realized another member of your family has compassion fatigue. It's really not hard to determine if you do or don't "have it." If you are currently a caregiver, you are probably experiencing compassion fatigue to a greater or lesser extent. So let's assume you have it! What now? Well, you need to practice some good self-care. Wait! I promise, no lame checklists of what you ought to do to regain the needed balance in your life. Instead, I have three suggestions for you to consider: be curious, be joyful, and be you.

Be Curious

How many times have you agreed to help someone without a thought? Someone calls and says, "Hey, I need a favor. Can you help?" You reflexively say, "Sure! What do you need?" Now let me ask you this.

Danger, Will Robinson

How do you typically respond to warnings? Do you stop at railroad crossings when the lights are flashing? Do you arise at the sound of your alarm clock? Does the timer on your stove generate action in the kitchen? In general, people are responsive to alarms and warnings. However, when approaching personal and professional boundaries, we often ignore the warnings. Word to the wise. Pay attention to your internal alarms. If something doesn't feel right, it's probably not. Danger, Will Robinson! You are about to cross a boundary! Proceed cautiously.

Perspiration

Why do we agree to do something before we know what is needed? Seems a little risky, doesn't it? But this is a common trait of caring, compassionate folks. We want to help, so we say "sure" before we know what we're getting into. This is often how compassion fatigue initiates and progresses. We say "yes" to all requests for help. We overextend and in the process experience overexposure to suffering.

So I invite you to consider a different response the next time someone asks for help. Be curious. Be inquisitive. Understand the parameters of the request: who, what, when, where, why, how, and for how long. Is this a short-

Not So Fast

The next time someone asks you for help, resist the temptation to immediately say "yes." Ask exactly what type of help the person is requesting and consider if you are able and willing to provide assistance. Curiosity may have killed the cat, but it just may save you from compassion fatigue!

Pure Genius!

or long-term commitment? What is your availability? Is this something you need, want, should, could, or have to do? After you have all the needed information, then make a thoughtful decision. And always remember, you can say "no." Being a kind and compassionate soul does not require an affirmative response to every request. Be curious. Be selective. Be well.

Be Joyful

Self-care. Such a lovely concept, yet so hard to do. And when experiencing compassion fatigue, self-care is particularly hard to accomplish. We already feel overwhelmed as it is. Don't add something else to my list of things to do! I know that's what you're thinking, right? So I won't suggest you go for a walk, write in a journal, take a bubble bath, or eat a lovely meal. Although those are all good things.

Inspiration

Sunrise, Sunset

How well I remember the morning of my mom's death. I recall little about the machines, the doctors, the sounds, or the smells of the hospital. What I remember is the incredible sunrise on that Easter morning. The subtle shades of pink, red, and coral provided a much-needed balm to my suffering soul. My mom died a short time later, and my memory will be forever colored by that glorious sunrise. My mom taught me well. She taught me how to see the sustaining grace in the ordinary moments of life. This appreciation and attentiveness to the moment, to the sacredness in the ordinary, sustained me the morning my mom died. As the sun set on my mom's life, I derived life-giving joy from a sublime sunrise.

Instead, I invite you to reflect on what gives you joy. Not happiness (which is fleeting). But sheer, unadulterated joy. Joy is the counterbalance to suffering. Suffering has the capacity to fill every fiber of our being. But, guess what? Joy works the same way. Being joyful is an intentional choice. We *seek* our sources of joy. So, what brings you joy? What fills you up? Lights you up? Sustains you during the toughest times?

I know from my experience and that of others, it's during the darkest times that our appreciation for the smallest mercies intensifies. We look for that glimmer of hope. And when we see that pin prick of light, we feel joyful! We don't have to look far, do we? If we are able to see the sacred in the ordinary, our lives will be forever filled with joy.

Be You

As caregivers, we can become consumed by what we do. We become the "role" and lose ourselves in the process. When caregiving dominates life, we are at great risk of experiencing compassion fatigue. Consequently, we need to find ways of moving in and out of that role on a daily basis. We need *transition rituals.* Transition rituals prepare us to move from one aspect of life to another, one role to another. The ritual serves to remind us that we are more than a job, more than a caregiver.

So, how do you shift gears and become just *you*? Listen to music on the drive home? Change clothes when you get home? Turn off your pager? Think about it. You can't be a caregiver 24/7 without compromising your own health and well-being. So implement a ritual that moves you from being a caregiver to being *you*. Then, on the flip side, implement a ritual

Transition Ritual Not Optional

When I come home from a conference or presentation, a transition ritual is *not* optional. As I cross the threshold, I am greeted by our herd of critters. They don't care where I've been or what I've been doing. Chaplain? Speaker? Writer? Caregiver? Nope. They recognize me as the human who loves, feeds, and plays with them. I am just Jane! And thank goodness for that. As the cats rub against my legs and the dog jumps up and down, I assume a different persona. I don't have to be *on*. I can just *be*. Critters are amazing, eh? Transition rituals are mandatory in our home. Thank goodness!

Inspiration

that helps you resume your role as caregiver. Be creative. Be innovative. You are limited only by your imagination when it comes to transition rituals.

Compassion fatigue is an inherent risk in caregiving. Because we are compassionate beings, we will experience this type of stress at some point. By understanding the source of compassion fatigue and being able to recognize the signs, we are better able to address our stress.

To Summarize...

🔍 Compassion fatigue is the overexposure to and/or overidentification with the suffering of another (people and animals).

🔍 As compassionate beings, we are emotionally moved by the suffering of others and desirous of *fixing* the situation. When situations cannot be *fixed*, we are at risk of experiencing compassion fatigue.

🔍 The signs of compassion fatigue are similar to other types of stress. Consequently, it is important to understand the source of compassion fatigue in order to mitigate the manifestations of this type of stress.

🔍 Once "diagnosed" with compassion fatigue, focus on being curious, being joyful, and being you. *Being* will serve you well!

Chapter 15

Resilience: Choosing to Bounce Back

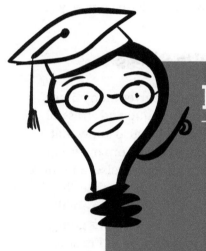

In This Chapter...

- How do we cope with stress?
- What are the basics of bounce?
- What are the common coping strategies and skills of resilient people?
- How can you learn to bounce in five minutes?

We've spent sufficient time highlighting the inherently stressful nature of caregiving. Caregiving is risky business, no doubt. But we need not be destroyed by the stress of the journey. So it's time to explore how we *choose* to deal with this stress. In **Chapter 3**, I introduced the concept of resilience. *Resilience* is a process of positive adaptation in the face of adversity. It enables us to bounce back from the blows of life and thus mitigate the stress generated by change and transition. An important process indeed!

In our discussion of resilience, I'll emphasize approaches, attitudes, beliefs, and actions that enable us to bounce back. Coping strategies and skills that facilitate the integration of change into our lives will be presented. It's important to note that how or if you choose to bounce is entirely up to you. We all bounce uniquely because we are unique individuals. However, there are consistent themes within the adaptive process of resilience worthy of consideration and review. Since resilience is not a trait, we can always learn new ways to bounce that ultimately serve us well. Being a lifelong student of bounce is, therefore, advisable.

If you're knee-deep in the caregiving journey, perhaps you're feeling a bit deflated. Maybe you've always been a bit underinflated? Whatever the reason, you just don't have much bounce! Well, I have a suggestion that will "pump you up!" Give me five minutes, and you'll be well on your way to bouncing higher than you ever imagined!

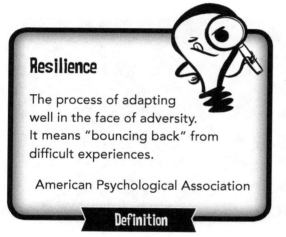

Resilience

The process of adapting well in the face of adversity. It means "bouncing back" from difficult experiences.

American Psychological Association

Definition

Coping with Stress

Having been a caregiver many times, I know how exhausting and stressful the journey can be. I also know that "helpful" suggestions from my friends of more sleep, more exercise, and more fun served only to infuriate me. Their comments indicated that they really didn't understand what I was going through. They didn't get it! I'm sure that's why I want to slap someone when I read the typical lists of caregiver stress suggestions. It's not that simple! There are times we *choose* to engage the caregiving process that goes against the grain. We *choose* to engage the journey of caregiving in a manner that actually increases our stress! We give too much. Do too much. Care too much. Or, perhaps, we don't show up. Don't care. Or can't care. As long as we understand the source of our stress and the risks associated with chronic stress, we are then responsible for managing our stress.

I am not going to tell you what you *must* or *should* do when it comes to caregiving and stress. It's your choice. We just need to go in with our eyes wide open. Caregiving *is* stressful. It is messy, nasty, tiring, frustrating, frightening, and downright *hard*! It is also meaningful, fulfilling, satisfying, glorious, and sacred. Caregiving is all that and so much more. So, have realistic expectations when it comes to caregiving and stress. You will be stressed. How you choose to deal with that stress is up to you.

How do we deal with all the changes and subsequent transitions posed by aging and illness? How do we handle the stress of uncertain times and destabilizing forces? In order to survive, we learn to cope. Utilizing a variety of strategies and skills, we attempt to resolve problems or adapt to various changes in life. The goal is to minimize stress. The manner in which we choose to cope determines whether we merely endure or truly engage the journey.

I've been singing the praises of proactive planning throughout this book. Prepare to care. This is a type of coping as well. If we can anticipate future needs, we certainly minimize the stress of aging and illness. Fewer fire drills. Less chaos. Less stress. Proactive planning reduces the size of the waves generated by change. Thus, we manage our stress and cope well.

However, we've admitted we aren't clairvoyant. Things will happen that we never imagined. Your mother has a stroke. Your dog is hit by a car. You fall down the stairs and break your leg. Wham! Life changes and stress rises. On those occasions, we must become adept at tap dancing for a period of time. We dance around assessing the situation. Asking questions. Gathering information. Identifying available resources. Developing a plan. Bottom line, we adapt to the change. We cope with the situation. And we consequently minimize the stress instigated by the unexpected change. Resilience is an effective process of adaptation. This process enables us to "bounce back" from adversity, loss, and suffering. Consequently, this is a process worthy of consideration by everyone on the caregiving journey.

Bouncing Across the Transitional Bridge

It's been a while since we discussed our image of change and transition—the bridge. This metaphor for change is central to the discussion of stress, coping, and resilience. So indulge me. Let's revisit the bridge and review the process of change one more time. I'll be referring to the image frequently for the rest of this chapter. If you know the bridge well, skip to the next section. I'll see you there.

A bridge reflects the process of change and transition quite well. Imagine yourself motoring through life. Things are going well. The path is level, until something happens. *Boom*! Something changes. Change is represented by a gateway, the entrance to a bridge. The bridge spans the space and time between what was (prior to change) and what will be (a new beginning). The transition, the aftermath of change, is the frightening time. *Bridge time.* Although the bridge transports you over the rough waters stirred up by the change in life, this is an incredibly stressful time.

Bridge time is a time of uncertainty. And as you know, uncertainty and unknowing breed stress. You strain to see what's on the other side of the bridge, to no avail. You attempt to assess the structural soundness of the bridge. You peer over the edge of the bridge and witness the churning waters caused by the change. And you wonder how in the world you landed on this bridge. Stressed? You bet!

Standing on the edge of the bridge, what are your options? In the words of Laurel and Hardy, "Well, here's another nice mess you've gotten us into!" Fighting back despair, you look around at the available options. Your first inclination is to turn around and make a mad dash back to "normal." But as you glance over your shoulder, you see a "Road Closed" sign. Can't go back. So you can either stand still, leap over the side, or move forward. What's it going to be? What do you choose to do? How do you make that decision?

Well, it all depends on how you choose to cope with the stress of the situation. If you're paralyzed by fear or tempted to take a flying leap off the bridge, please consider another option before finalizing your plans. Don't let the fear of change and transition be the determining factor of what happens next. Instead, consider *bouncing* across the bridge. Yep. Bouncing! I think you'll find the process of resilience to be an effective way to transition to the other side of the bridge. Resilience actually facilitates the integration of change into your life. Imagine resilience as the conveyor belt on the bridge of transition, moving you from one side to the other. From what was to what will be. Bouncing is an amazingly effective way to transition. Keep reading.

Amazing Examples of Resilience

- Viktor Frankl: Following a three-year internment in the Nazi concentration camps of World War II, Frankl founded the Third Viennese School of Psychotherapy and taught a generation about the importance of meaning.

- Hiroshima: Two weeks following the atomic bomb blast in 1945, banks reopened. One month later, people started moving back into the city. After three months, the city achieved a population of 33 percent of the prebomb population (as noted by George Bonanno, *The Other Side of Sadness*, 2009).

- Vietnam Prisoners of War (POWs): Many POWs reported an enhanced appreciation of life, strengthened relationships, and a renewed sense of meaning and purpose because of their war experience (as reported by Steven Southwick, 2012).

Example

Basics of Bounce

I marvel at the human capacity to bounce back from adversity. Don't you? How do people survive experiences such as the Holocaust, 9/11, Hiroshima, internment, Alzheimer's disease, and Hurricane Sandy? It's more than a question of survival. How do people live to thrive beyond the experience of profound suffering and loss? How are they able to bounce back? Resilience. What does it mean to be resilient? You bend, but you don't break! *The Road to Resilience* is described by the American Psychological Association on its website (apa.org/helpcenter/road-resilience.aspx). Additionally, Dr. Steven Southwick explores the factors that contribute to resilience in his book *Resilience: The Science of Mastering Life's Greatest Challenges* (2012). Both sources identify the fundamental building blocks of resilience recognized in people who bounce back from adversity. These are the same building blocks—the attitudes, thoughts, and behaviors—I have witnessed in resilient family members, friends, colleagues, and clients. Combining my personal observations with the work of others, we'll continue to explore the process of resilience.

Resilience is a process of adaptation to adverse conditions. It is not a trait. Not something you're born with. Instead, resilience includes attitudes, thoughts, behaviors, and actions that can be learned (or enhanced) at any time. Basically, coping strategies and skills. It's also good to know that resilience is quite common. In fact, it is the norm rather than the exception. And yet we are always amazed by the bounce that others demonstrate in the midst of daunting situations. I'm sure you've been amazed at your own ability to bounce during a crisis. The option to bounce across the transitional bridge is a viable option for all of us. However, it doesn't just happen. Bouncing is an intentional choice. We *choose* to bounce.

It's also important to realize that resilience is rooted in realism. Bouncing requires an honest assessment of the situation. We must see life as it is, not as we wish it to be. Based on a realistic assessment, we then make a conscious choice in how to respond to the challenge. Yes, resilience requires an optimistic approach. However, optimism tempered with realism is an essential key to bouncing back from adversity. Don't bring your rose-colored glasses to the bridge. To bounce well, you need a clear, unfiltered view of the bridge.

Coping Strategies and Skills of Resilient People

What does it take to bounce? There is no simple answer to that question. People bounce for a variety of reasons and in a variety of ways. However, there are some common coping skills shared by people who bounce well that we'll discuss. You may identify with some of the elements of resilience, but not all. It would be a rare person, indeed, who possessed all the coping strategies and skills noted. So recognize your current strengths and leverage them. Then identify attitudes, approaches, and behaviors that could provide an even bigger bounce. Remember, resilience is something we learn and develop over a lifetime. We always have the opportunity to develop new coping strategies and skills. Sometimes we are forced into action in order to bounce across the transitional bridge. Attentiveness to our bouncing ability serves us well. Just like checking the air in your tires, do a personal pressure check from time to time. So let's consider the various coping strategies and skills employed by resilient people. What do we need to bounce well?

Sense of Meaning and Purpose

According to Viktor Frankl, the driving force for humanity is the search for meaning. We need to understand the "whys" of life. Meaning and purpose motivate us to persist, to bounce across transitional bridges. Without meaning, why bother? With meaning, people are capable of extraordinary things. According to Friedrich Nietzsche, a nineteenth-century existentialist, "He who has a *why* to live can bear almost any *how*." This sentiment has been proven to be true time and time again. Read the memoirs of Holocaust survivors. Examine the biographies of Vietnam POWs. When people believe there is a meaning and purpose in life (the why), they are able to endure the most brutal conditions.

Now reflect on your experience of caregiving. Aren't there moments when you desperately need and want answers? Meaning is essential for all persons, in all times, and in all places. Meaning and purpose motivate us to bounce across the transitional bridge. What is the meaning that supports and sustains you? What is the "why" of your life? Important to consider and determine.

Faith

During the most challenging times of life, our day-to-day coping strategies and skills often prove to be inadequate. When we are literally brought to our knees by life, we rely on our foundational beliefs to support and sustain us. In **Chapter 9**, we discussed the concepts of religion and spirituality. Since everyone has a unique understanding of those terms, I opted to call our sustaining and guiding beliefs "faith." Call it what you will; our faith guides and sustains us during the times that try our souls.

Furthermore, the practice of our faith—the rituals—serves to connect us to meaning, purpose, community, our sense of the sacred, and hope. This particular coping strategy is inextricably tied to the previous strategy, meaning and purpose. Regardless of your particular faith tradition, the function of faith is to facilitate the search for meaning. The search for significance in this life. I have yet to read an account of extraordinary adversity that doesn't include a discussion of the sustaining attributes of faith. Apparently, being faithful benefits our ability to bounce.

Optimism

How do you see life? Do you tend to focus on the positive or negative aspects of life? We all have a natural tendency to see the world as either a half-full or a half-empty glass. It's important to understand our preferred perspective since it informs our ability to bounce. Optimism, realistic optimism, is fundamental to resilience. For example, if you look across the transitional bridge and lament that all is lost, why would you choose to bounce across? What's the point? An optimist, on the other hand, looks across the bridge and sees opportunity and visualizes possibilities. Optimists do not allow adversity to dominate the view. Optimists see beyond the current malaise and imagine better times ahead.

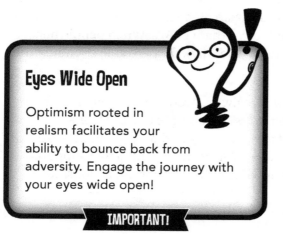

Eyes Wide Open

Optimism rooted in realism facilitates your ability to bounce back from adversity. Engage the journey with your eyes wide open!

IMPORTANT!

By realistically assessing the situation, the optimist engages in productive problem solving. One step at a time, the optimist figures out how to move from one side of the bridge to the other. The future-focused optimist sees beyond the frightening transitional bridge and chooses to bounce toward the alluring possibilities on the other side. Quite often, the optimist's bounce is fueled by a foundational, sustaining faith. Are you starting to see how the themes of resilience, the coping strategies and skills, are related? Keep reading. The plot thickens.

Courage

Courage is required to navigate the caregiving journey well. Around every bend in the road, we encounter challenging and frightening aspects of aging and illness. Uncertainty. Unknowing. The specter of death. Pain. Disability. Loss. Continuous change. A myriad of things that can potentially intimidate, threaten, and frighten us. In the absence of courage, we'd be paralyzed by fear. Standing at the edge of the bridge, unable to contemplate the needed crossing to continue on with life. In the absence of courage, fear disables us.

How do we overcome fear? Knowledge. Knowledge is power—one of my mantras. We must know what we're up against in order to move through and live beyond our fears. Knowledge addresses the fear of the unknown and initiates a cascade of other coping strategies and skills. Knowledge leads to

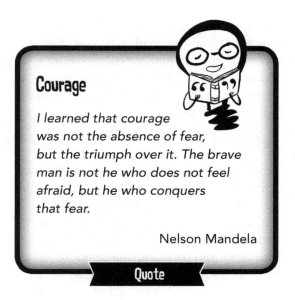

Courage

I learned that courage was not the absence of fear, but the triumph over it. The brave man is not he who does not feel afraid, but he who conquers that fear.

Nelson Mandela

Quote

confidence. Confidence naturally feeds an optimistic perspective. Optimism is sustained by foundational faith. And faith provides the motivational meaning and purpose to bounce across the bridge. Be brave. Be bold. *Bounce!*

Respond to Life

If you haven't figured out by now, I feel compelled to tell you: you can't control everything that happens in life. No matter how hard you try, things happen that you don't anticipate, don't want, and don't like. That's life. So it does little good to stand at the gateway to the bridge bemoaning your fate in life. Granted, we all take a time out now and then to have a major pity party. But, eventually, we crawl out of our pit of despair to evaluate the situation. We may not like it, but we have a responsibility to respond to life.

Furthermore, the implications of our responses radiate throughout the system in which we live. Remember our discussion of systems theory? We are all interconnected. So whatever we choose to do in response to life will impact the entire system to a greater or lesser extent. In the context of caregiving, our families are directly affected by the choices we make.

Additionally, the attitude we assume in response to life has direct implications on the choices we make. Optimistic? Pessimistic? Angry? Despairing? Resentful? Our attitude colors our judgment. So, before acting, we need to consider the consequences of our actions. How will others be affected? Positively? Negatively? Remember, we must bounce responsibly!

Self-Confidence and Self-Knowing

When the winds of change howl, we need an anchor in the storm. We need a sense of who we are and what we are about in order to cope with the challenges of life. Self-confidence. Guiding values and principles. These are the anchors that hold us steady in the roughest waters. When everything

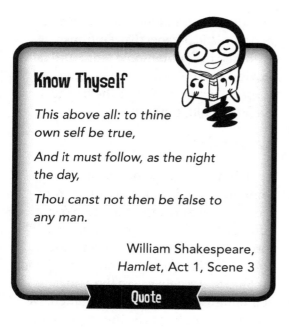

Know Thyself

This above all: to thine own self be true,

And it must follow, as the night the day,

Thou canst not then be false to any man.

William Shakespeare,
Hamlet, Act 1, Scene 3

Quote

else looks unfamiliar and menacing on the transitional bridge, look within to regain the needed confidence and calm to proceed. Bouncing benefits from self-confidence and adherence to personal values.

Community

Life is not a solo flight. As we wing our way through life, we rely on family and friends. And, they rely on us. Interdependence is not a sign of weakness. Rather, these mutually beneficial relationships reflect a healthy and robust social support system. Our social networks provide vital support, especially during times of trial and tribulation. In fact, interdependence provides a foundation for resilience. When dealing with long-term caregiving concerns, families can often feel isolated and alone. When doing "bridge time," we need our supportive and sustaining relationships. In order to thrive—in order to bounce—we need other people. Bouncing is an individual choice. But it never hurts to have a few cheerleaders urging us on.

Resilient Role Models

Resilience is not a trait we inherit. Rather, it is a process we learn and develop over the course of a lifetime. And, as is often the case, the best way to learn is by observing. In **Chapter 3**, I shared the story of my mom bouncing in the Grand Canyon. I am sure you know people who demonstrate the ability to bounce as well. People who bend but don't break. People who bounce back from the blows of life, seemingly bigger and better than ever. Identify the resilient role models in your life and follow their lead. You'll be bouncing across the bridge before you know it!

Physical, Emotional, and Mental Fitness

Physical, emotional, and mental fitness enhance our ability to bounce. Hence, we are wise to engage in activities that exercise the mind, body, and spirit.

Be Observant

Like a picture, a role model is worth a thousand words. Instead of reading about resilience, watch someone bounce. Look around. I am sure there is someone in your world who has bouncing down to a fine art. Observe carefully.

Perspiration

During times of tremendous stress, physical exercise is often a lifesaver on many levels. Exercise results not only in physical fitness but also in emotional and mental fitness. Physically, exercise serves to counteract the negative health implications of chronic stress (compromised immune system). Emotionally, exercise results in the production of endorphins that generate a sense of well-being. And mentally, exercise enhances self-confidence and reduces stress.

Mindfulness meditation also enhances emotional fitness. The goal is to achieve a sense of stability and calm. Something we all need in the midst of crisis and chaos, right? You might opt to engage in some of the traditional meditation practices of specific faith traditions such as Buddhism or Christianity (centering prayer). Or be creative. Develop a meditation practice that serves you well—practice being the operative term. Commit to faithfully practicing your mode of meditation by reserving a specific time or times of the day for contemplation. You might also consider designating a particular place in your home as meditative space. Or, if you prefer, enjoy your meditative time outdoors. To determine what works best for you, experiment with silence, music, readings, and motion. Be creative! Design a meditative practice that suits your personality and allows you to be present to the moment.

Mental fitness during stressful times is incredibly important as well. If mentally sharp, we are better able to focus, problem solve, and make decisions. So consider engaging in activities that are enjoyable but also stretch your cognitive abilities. Crossword puzzles. Sudoku. Learn a new language. Play an instrument. The activities will prepare you well for the bridge. If you want to bounce higher and faster, get mentally fit!

Cognitive Flexibility

Being rigid rarely serves us well. In fact, it is impossible to be resilient—to bounce—if we are rigid. By definition, resilient means to bend, not break.

Meditation in Motion

The first year I attended seminary, I was determined to learn the practice of centering prayer. I had several friends who were quite keen on the practice. So I thought it advisable to learn the process. I must admit, I failed miserably. Try as I might, the practice served to stress me out rather than focus and calm my mind. So I developed a practice that serves me quite well. Meditation in motion. When I walk, cycle, or hike, those are the times I feel the most calm and most connected to that which I deem sacred. So, if the traditional meditation practices don't serve you well—get moving! My pedal and pray time is the best!

Inspiration

This applies to our physical, emotional, spiritual, and cognitive demeanor. Cognitively, change is difficult to wrap our minds around when it is unexpected or unwanted. We obsess on what *should* be instead of what is. Recognition of what is within our control and what is not enhances cognitive flexibility. When life changes, we must be willing to think about life in a different way. The game changed. Our expectations must change as well.

Humor

Let's get serious. Life is no laughing matter. Every day, countless stories of suffering, destruction, and tragedy bombard us. We witness family and friends challenged by advanced age and serious illness. Sometimes, it's just too much! And then, one more stressful thing occurs, and . . . we *laugh!* Things get *so* bad that we *have* to laugh. This is the blessing of laughter. It's a fabulous way to cope with the tension and stress of change and transition. So keep a sense of humor. We can giggle as we bounce across the bridge.

Accept Change as the Norm

In **Chapter 3**, we discussed the fact that life is a continuous process of change. Change *is* the norm. Yet we live as if change is an aberration. Our resistance to change inhibits our ability to bounce. Instead of looking across the transitional bridge, we long to return to "normal." Eventually, the reality comes to bear, and we begrudgingly inch forward. We make life so hard, don't we? We would save ourselves significant time, effort, and suffering if we were to accept change as the norm and bounce across the bridge. Let it be so!

Survivor versus Victim Mentality

Resilience is an intentional choice. Whether we bounce or not hinges on how we see ourselves. Victim or survivor? Victims are deflated by the circumstances of life. Everything is hard. Life is unjust. Everything is beyond control! Victims, therefore, lack the courage, motivation, and desire to bounce across the transitional bridge. Victims experience a life of unending, oppressive stress. Survivors, on the other hand, know well the twists and turns of life. Yet survivors opt to visualize a life beyond the bridge. Survivors seek meaning in the midst of the chaos and crisis. Survivors have the confidence and the courage to bounce across the bridge. Victim or survivor? The choice is ours to make, and the ensuing life is ours to live. Choose wisely.

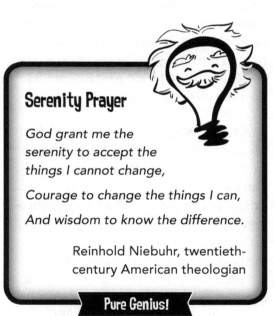

Serenity Prayer

God grant me the serenity to accept the things I cannot change,

Courage to change the things I can,

And wisdom to know the difference.

Reinhold Niebuhr, twentieth-century American theologian

Pure Genius!

Gratitude for Growth

Whether we like it or not, it's the darkest days that offer the greatest opportunities for growth. Think about it. When things are going well and life is grand, there is no need to question, seek, and explore. There is no reason to push beyond the edges of the known existence. What's the point? Life is grand. Enjoy! It's the dark nights of the soul that demand our attention. Rattle our cages. Shake the foundation on which we stand. And threaten to destroy our sense of self. In the darkness, our mettle is tested, our faith questioned, and our essence exposed.

Not a pleasant experience by any means! But with enough time and distance, we recognize the gift of darkness: growth. The hard times in life force us to grow in ways previously unimagined. If we choose to be resilient—bouncing back from adversity—we'll eventually learn to be grateful for the growth derived from our efforts.

A Funny Funeral

I have attended a number of funerals over the course of my lifetime. Each one unique. However, there is one funeral that stands out in my mind because it was so incredibly *funny*. The woman who died was a beloved member of her family and community. She was known for having a raucous sense of humor. Evidently, it was a gift shared by her entire family. At her funeral, all of her siblings regaled us with stories about the deceased. Yes, poignant, loving tales that brought tears to our eyes as we laughed hysterically! The laughter did not diminish our sense of loss, but instead helped us cope with a tremendous void that remains even today. Humor enabled all of us to bounce out of the church and get on with life. I am sure the deceased had a good laugh as well. That's how she bounced!

Pure Genius!

Five-Minute Plan—The Beginning of Bounce

Are you starting to feel less stressed? I would certainly hope so! Knowing the basics of resilience, you can bounce over the challenges of aging and illness with your eyes shut, right? You're pumped up to one hundred pounds, and you're capable of bouncing back from the blows of life. Bring it on! Oh, am I sensing a bit of trepidation? Are you not sure how to start bouncing? Well, let's see if I can provide the little push that you need.

Several years ago, a woman approached me at the conclusion of a caregiving workshop. She herself was a caregiver and highly complimentary of the program. However, she had a suggestion regarding the section on caregiver stress. Although the ideas shared were viable, the options were not possible for this woman. She didn't have time for a walk, a movie, or lunch with a friend (most caregivers don't!). When asked about her caregiving situation, she calmly explained the following. She was the primary caregiver for her husband who had Alzheimer's disease. She also cared for her son diagnosed with a congenital, cognitive disability. Her mother had been diagnosed with pancreatic cancer three weeks before the workshop and would be moving in shortly. And this woman worked full time because her family needed the income and health care benefits. Obviously, time was a priceless commodity in her world.

As I listened in total amazement, I wondered how this woman was able to make a complete sentence, remain vertical, and radiate a sense of optimism and positivity. I marveled at her composure and attitude. So I asked her how she did it. What was her secret? That's when she shared her suggestion about caregiver stress.

It does no good to recommend options for stress relief that are unattainable to stressed-out caregivers. Sure, a massage would be lovely. But when? So any suggestion must be enjoyable *and* possible. In her current situation, she practiced the Five Minute Plan of stress relief. She explained it this way. Every morning at 8:00, she went into the only room in her house that locked, her bathroom. She lowered the seat on her throne and sat down. She then selected the songs of the day from her iPod, cranked it up, and reveled in the music for five minutes. At the end of five minutes, she turned off the music. She arose from her throne. Looked in the mirror and said, "Get out there. You can do this one more day." And with that, she opened the door and reengaged her journey. One step at a time.

This is the beginning of bounce. This is actually the essence of bounce. Confidence. Faith. Purpose. Courage. Optimism. Start with five minutes. We can all find five minutes in a day. Do something that fills you up, lifts you up, and sustains you for the next twenty-three hours and fifty-five minutes. Then do it again. As you become accustomed to this ritual of self-care, I encourage you to extend the time from five to ten minutes. Then ten to fifteen. To bounce well, we must practice, practice, practice.

To Summarize...

- Caregiving is stressful. No doubt about it. However, we need not be destroyed by stress. Instead, we need to effectively cope with the stress. *Resilience* is a process of positive adaptation in the face of adversity. It enables us to bounce back from the blows of life and thus mitigate the stress generated by change and transition. An important process indeed!

- Resilience is not a trait. Rather, resilience involves behaviors, attitudes, actions, and thoughts that can be learned and developed. Although each person responds to adversity uniquely, there are recognizable themes found in resilient people.

- Resilience is a process that enables and empowers caregivers and care receivers to navigate the daunting transitions prompted by change. When resilient, the burdens of caregiving may bend us, but we will not break. We will bounce back. We will be changed, and we will be able to continue the journey.

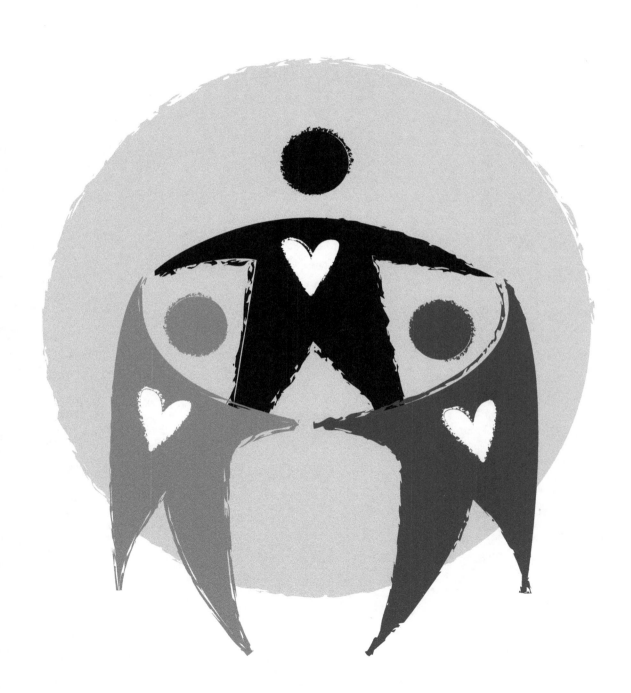

The Philosophy of Collaborative Care

Over the past decade, I have created and presented numerous caregiving workshops and programs for families and health care professionals. I spent concerted time and effort attempting to convince individuals that it was okay to ask for and to receive help from family, friends, and professionals. However, the majority of people I encountered opted to remain as the primary caregiver or to enlist the help of a select few. In an attempt to understand the pervasive resistance to creating teams or communities of care, I chatted with caregivers and care receivers in order to identify the points of resistance. I'll share the wisdom so graciously offered by those caregivers and care receivers. Whether you choose to serve as a primary caregiver or opt to organize a caregiving team, a collaborative approach to care benefits everyone involved in the journey of caregiving.

Chapter 16

May I Help You?

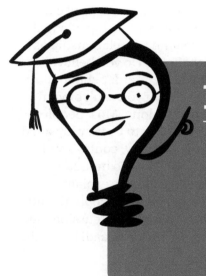

In This Chapter...

- Why doesn't one size fit all when it comes to caregiving?
- What does resistance to assistance look like?
- What is caregiving like on Venus and Mars?
- How can the relationship between shepherd and sheep inform the journey of caregiving?

A t some point in the caregiving journey, we all need help. But for most of us, it's hard to ask. How can we overcome our resistance to assistance? When I worked as a palliative care educator, I became enamored with a team model of caregiving designed to address this issue. I appreciated the potential benefits of sharing the responsibilities of caregiving, having served as a primary caregiver. Although the team approach works well for some families, there are other options worthy of consideration. One size does *not* fit all!

Whether caregivers and care receivers opt to accept needed help from others depends on a variety of factors. Certainly, family and cultural norms are

May I Help You?

I often ask those attending programs on caregiving if they easily ask for help. Not surprisingly, only a few people profess to routinely ask others for help. The rest of us resist asking for and accepting help. How about you? May I help you? If this simple question causes you to squirm in your chair, break out in a sweat, or run for the hills, perhaps you have a resistance to assistance as well! Now is your opportunity to discover the roots of your resistance. Keep reading!

IMPORTANT!

important considerations. But there are other important issues that influence our ability and willingness to accept help. Knowing the possible points of resistance allows for respectful and beneficial discussions regarding caregiving options.

Our experience of caregiving, whether as caregiver or care receiver, is influenced by our understanding of the relationship between the giver and receiver of care. Do you view this as a relationship of equals? Do you understand the relationship as mutually beneficial? Do you believe caregiving to be an interdependent relationship? Well, if you can't or you don't, you are not alone. Most people view the relationship to be very lopsided regarding responsibility, control, and contribution. So I hope to broaden your view of caregiving by explaining the relationship between shepherd and sheep. It can be a woolly discussion, but I promise it won't be all baaad! Just wait. *Ewe* will see!

One Size Does *Not* Fit All

In **Chapter 1**, we reviewed the daunting statistics related to caregiving in the United States today. Obviously, caregiving is not a role to assume casually. As primary caregivers, we risk compromising our own health and well-being over the course of the journey if we overextend ourselves physically, emotionally, spiritually, and financially. So, we are wise to consider the available options for fulfilling the role of caregiver. Who is available to help? Who can we ask for help? How do we choose to engage the journey of caregiving? Here are some options to consider:

 Primary caregiver (Lone Ranger model). Primary caregivers assume the responsibility for the majority of caregiving needs. Although this model of caregiving can take a tremendous toll on the primary caregiver, it is the model of choice for many families.

💡 Primary caregiver with backup. Primary caregivers may opt to recruit a family member or friend to occasionally "fill in" when respite is needed or wanted. This option allows the primary caregiver the time to refresh, renew, and rest periodically. It also provides a sense of security for the caregiver and care receiver. Just in case something happens to the primary caregiver, there is someone waiting in the wings to step in and assume the responsibilities of care.

💡 Primary caregiver with family assistance. Primary caregivers may choose to coordinate caregiving responsibilities with family members, sharing in the responsibilities of care on a regular basis. This model works well for families living in the same area. For those families that are geographically dispersed, some duties of caregiving can still be shared through the use of technology.

💡 Primary caregiver with team assistance. Primary caregivers may choose to coordinate caregiving responsibilities with family members, friends, colleagues, and others who volunteer for various caregiving tasks. The team approach to care requires an initial, concerted effort to coordinate care. If done well, the caregiving team can serve the family incredibly well. However, the majority of families find this process overwhelming and opt for a different model of caregiving.

When I began researching the various models of caregiving ten years ago, I knew the tremendous risk primary caregivers assumed. I had experienced the stress of primary caregiving multiple times caring for family members. Hence, the concept of sharing the responsibility of care appealed to me. I developed a comprehensive training program for caregivers with the goal of empowering individuals and families alike to create caregiving teams. The workshops were well attended. The concept and training materials well received. However, few caregiving

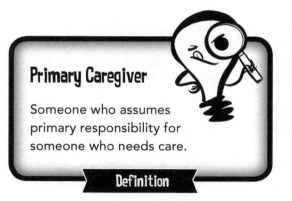

Primary Caregiver

Someone who assumes primary responsibility for someone who needs care.

Definition

teams resulted as a consequence of the training efforts. As you might imagine, I was disappointed and somewhat perplexed. The team approach to caregiving made so much sense! However, this wasn't the first hypothesis to fail the litmus test in the trenches of reality.

In order to identify the disconnect between hypothesis and reality, I interviewed numerous caregivers and care receivers. Why was a potentially beneficial model of caregiving rejected by most families? I spoke with families that used the team approach and those that didn't. The honest assessment of the model served to enrich my understanding of the caregiving process.

The experience for those individuals or families using a caregiving team was generally positive. However, the primary caregivers reflected that the idea of asking others for help was difficult, if not impossible. So the teams were assembled by people other than the primary caregiver. In fact, some teams were formed despite the primary caregiver's objection or without their initial consent. Friends created the team and showed up! The primary caregiver was given little option but to accept the help of the team. After the fact, the primary caregivers were incredibly thankful for the additional help, singing the praises of various team members. Yet, without exception, the primary caregivers said they would never have created a caregiving team on their own. They needed that extra push and directive from other family members and friends.

The majority of families interviewed did not seek help beyond the inner circle of family and friends. When asked about the caregiving team option, the families helped identify important stumbling blocks for this team model of caregiving:

- Initial team formation required too much time and effort.

- The family or person had no potential team members.

- The process seemed too complicated.

- The family was already overwhelmed. They didn't want one more thing to do.

- The resistance to ask for assistance was too strong to overcome.

Although the foundational logic of caregiving teams is sound, the model of team caregiving is not easily embraced or implemented by the majority of people in the United States. That is the reality. So instead of stubbornly fighting the strong headwind of caregiver resistance, I opted to ride the jet stream of public consensus. Even if the team model of caregiving makes sense, people will not use it if they don't want it, trust it, or like it. So instead of force fitting every family into the caregiving team model, I invite families to consider all the available options. To understand the benefits and risks of each approach. And to identify the approach to caregiving that meets the needs, wants, and norms of the family. Granted, the selected mode of operation may not be the most logical or beneficial for the caregiver and/or care receiver. But caregiving isn't always logical! Emotions, personal preferences, and resistance to assistance often trump logic when it comes to caregiving.

Natural-Born Care Receivers

It's interesting to realize that human beings are born as natural care receivers. Think about it. Did you routinely reject clean diapers and bottles? I doubt it. Babies know how to graciously receive care. Out of the mouths of babes...

Pure Genius!

Points of Resistance

Resistance to assistance can be an issue, whether forming a caregiving team or asking another family member for help. What are the roots of resistance over which so many of us stumble? Working with families confronted by the challenges of caregiving over the past decade, I have identified consistent themes of resistance. Perhaps you will resonate with some of these points of resistance.

Denial

Caregivers often deny feeling overwhelmed and exhausted. For some, it seems inappropriate to complain since the people for whom they care have progressive or life-limiting illnesses. In comparison, being a caregiver is not so bad! Thus, the caregivers deny needing or wanting additional help.

Not Going There!

If someone slams a door in your face, you aren't apt to knock again. It's amazing how the sound of that slamming door echoes throughout a lifetime. In fact, the sound can be so loud as to inhibit our ability to ask for needed help. I met a woman years ago who was overwhelmed by the demands of life and caregiving. Three children. Work. Home. And a severely compromised husband due to a traumatic brain injury. As we discussed her situation, I asked if her mother would be able and willing to assist. Without hesitation, the woman said, "Not going there!" She was so resolute in her response that I knew there was more to the story. And there was. Many years before, she had asked her mother for help with one of the children. Her mother refused to help. *Wham!* Door shut. Although the woman now desperately needed help with her husband, she wasn't going to risk being rejected once again by her mother. She refused to go there. The fear of rejection overshadowed her need for help.

Uninspired

Pride

Many caregivers assume the role because of family expectations, cultural norms, or personal responsibility. Being a competent, capable caregiver is a source of pride. To request or accept help would be a perceived failing on the part of the caregiver and a source of humiliation and/or shame.

Fear of Rejection

Although many caregivers recognize the need for additional help, they fear being rejected by those asked to help. Everyone is so incredibly busy. Who has time to help? It's safer for caregivers to keep doing what they're doing and avoid the possibility of rejection.

Lack of Information (about the Disease Process)

Once again, let me stress the importance of knowledge. Knowledge about the disease process and anticipated caregiving needs is vitally important for families to meet the challenges of caregiving. Knowing what to expect enables caregivers to proactively plan for additional assistance as the care receiver's condition worsens. When relying on family and friends for the additional support, adequate lead time can make the difference between a positive and negative response to a request for help.

Cultural and Family Norms

In **Chapter 5**, we discussed how family legacies of care and cultural norms influence how we engage the journey of caregiving. The probability of outside assistance with care is highly unlikely if the expectation within the family is that family cares for family. Additionally, there may be norms as to who serves as the primary caregiver. If so, the majority of caregiving responsibilities may land on the shoulders of one person within the family. This can weigh one person down over an extended period of time.

Privacy/Secrecy

Is your family system open or closed? Closed families appear to be private or even secretive, thus limiting the ability for personal and professional caregivers to assist with caregiving needs. Sometimes the secretive nature of a family is related to a family history of abuse and/or addiction.

Example

That's Not How You Load a Dishwasher

I could tell Rachel needed to rest. She was recovering from major surgery. Although doing well, she tired quickly. So I suggested she take a nap while I cleaned the kitchen and started dinner for her family. As I was loading the dishwasher, Rachel's husband returned from the grocery store with bags in hand. Jim had been covering all the bases since Rachel's surgery, and I could tell he was a bit weary. However, Jim was not comfortable accepting help from Rachel's friends. In fact, this was the first time he had allowed me to fill in while he ran errands. As I was about to shut the dishwasher, he leaned over my shoulder and said, "That's not how you load a dishwasher." After which, he proceeded to right the wrong and moved dishes into the proper places. At first, I thought he was kidding. But no! He was serious. As he feverishly juggled dishes, I became somewhat apprehensive about his assessment of my culinary skills. As it turned out, Jim declined my subsequent offers to help. To this day, I don't know if it was the dishes or my lasagna that was the deal breaker.

Control

We often resist asking for or accepting help from others because we refuse to relinquish even a little bit of control. Although there is no one right way to do anything, we think there is. *My* way! So, as caregivers, we perceive ourselves to be irreplaceable. The need to control everything often proves to be the Achilles' heel of caregivers. If we are able to loosen our grip on the joystick of life, others will then be able to assist us in meaningful ways.

Isolation

Currently, the journey of caregiving averages 4.6 years. Over the course of the journey, caregivers and care receivers can become isolated from other family members and friends. As social connections weaken or fade away, caregivers and care receivers become even more reluctant to ask for help. In the case of advanced age, the care receiver may outlive other family and friends. As the last person standing, there is no one to ask for help. In cases of extreme isolation, volunteers can be recruited to fill in some of the gaps of care.

Lack of Role Recognition

In some instances, caregivers refuse to ask for help because they don't identify with the role of caregiver. This lack of role recognition happens quite often in the case of spousal care. The person providing care understands the additional responsibilities as part of the role of husband or wife. The person vowed to provide this care. Hence, it is inappropriate to ask others for help.

For most of us, it's not easy to ask for help. But if we understand the "why" beneath our reluctance, perhaps we can overcome our resistance to assistance. Ultimately, it's a choice. I'm not saying you should, must, have to, ought to, or need to ask others for help. But if you *choose* to ask for or receive help from others, you will probably encounter a sharp point of resistance somewhere along the way. Better to know the location of that sharp point than to step on it unexpectedly. As always, knowledge is power. Watch your step!

Needs Versus Wants

At the end of the day, as either caregiver or care receiver, we may *know* that additional assistance is advisable. We *know* it, but we don't *want* it.

For whatever reason, we are resistant. And unless or until there is a crisis mandating additional help, we'll tolerate the situation because that's what we want. In **Chapter 17**, we'll explore how our resistance to assistance changes once a tipping point is encountered. This is the moment when *needs* trump *wants*. Additional assistance is no longer optional due to safety or health concerns.

If asking for help is hard for you, please know I feel your pain! Several years ago, I had a conversation with a dear friend and colleague about the concept of caregiving teams. She turned the tables when she asked, "Would you want a caregiving team?" The question took me by surprise. It was easy to sing the praises of sharing the responsibilities of care to other people. But what about me? What about my family? I found myself tripping over my family norm of primary caregiving. I know that model so well. It's my comfort zone. So, like you, I'll continue to bump into my points of resistance when it comes to asking for help. But that doesn't preclude the possibility of transformation. Different times and different challenges often require different responses. At every turn, we have the opportunity to learn and to grow in amazing ways. Being open to possibility is one of the best ways to counter resistance. Never say never!

Would You?

There are many viable caregiving options and approaches worthy of consideration. Before promoting a particular model of caregiving to other people (your family, friends, and/or clients), ask yourself *the* important question. Is this something you would want if you were the care receiver? Would you embrace this model of care as the caregiver?

Inspiration

Differences in Caregiving on Mars and Venus

Caregiving is becoming gender neutral. Both men and women serve as caregivers. In the United States, it's estimated that 60 percent of caregivers are women, 40 percent are men. These numbers reflect how people self-report. So, if a person doesn't perceive the role as caregiver, it's not reported as such. Quite often, men don't see themselves as caregivers. Rather, the role is that of son, husband, or partner. So, it's important to understand that men and women engage and perceive the role of caregiver differently. It's not about being right or wrong. It's just different. These differences often determine the caregiver's willingness to seek assistance or accept help from others.

Let's compare and contrast the journey of caregiving on Mars and Venus. Although I'm not a fan of stereotypes, there are basic, fundamental differences in how men and women engage life. For example, there are extensive studies documenting the differences in communication and decision-making styles between men and women. These gender-specific tendencies influence how men and women serve as caregivers. So please accept the following comments with an open mind and accepting heart. You may not be the stereotypical man or woman. But you probably know one! So consider how men and women typically differ in the following aspects and the implications those differences have in regard to caregiving. The goal is to recognize and honor the differences so we can help each other along the way.

Social Support

Women derive needed and desired social support from girlfriends. We count on our gal pals to support and sustain us through good times and bad. Consequently, as caregivers, women have an established network of friends to discuss, debate, and process the questions and concerns of the journey. In contrast, men typically derive social support from a life partner. Men don't have the expansive social network that most women do. Hence, as caregivers, men often feel more isolated than women. Knowing this, instead of waiting for men to ask for help, perhaps we can be more proactive in offering assistance.

Communication Styles

Women communicate to establish and reinforce relationships, whereas men communicate to convey facts. Hence, women share facts as well as feelings. Since caregiving is an emotional roller coaster, caregivers (male and female) experience a myriad of emotions that can build up over time if not expressed or addressed. An inability or unwillingness to articulate these emotions often leads to serious issues of depression for caregivers. So pay attention to communication styles. We can't force people to communicate. But we can create a safe space in which people feel invited to share. We can offer to listen. Whether male or female caregiver, this is a tremendous gift indeed.

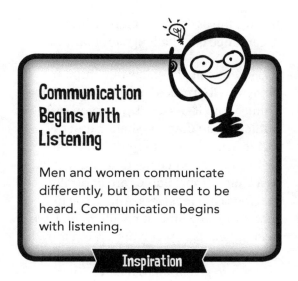

Decision Making

Women are known for building consensus, while men are known for being directive and autonomous when it comes to decision making. Could this have implications on how the journey of caregiving unfolds? *Absolutely*! There are times that demand quick, authoritative decision making. In the midst of a crisis, we don't have the luxury of time to make sure everyone is on the same page. However, there are other times when families need to take the time to discuss, debate, and build consensus. Both styles of decision making are needed in the context of caregiving. The challenge is to find a happy medium that serves the caregiver, the care receiver, and the family well.

Role Identification

Men and women relate to the role of caregiver quite differently. This is due partly to the stereotypical female image of "caregiver" in the United States. Women assume the role naturally due to nature, nurture, and societal expectations. Women identify with the role, whereas most men do not. Instead, men will describe their role as that of husband, son, brother, friend, or partner. Consequently, men may not identify with the term "caregiver." In order to effectively communicate with and assist a caregiver, we must first establish how the person self-defines. Then we can use language that will resonate with the person.

The Quintessential Model of Interdependence

Basic to our ability and willingness to ask for and receive help is our understanding of the caregiving roles—caregiver versus care receiver. If we perceive being a care receiver as something less than desirable, we will be reluctant to assume, accept, and fulfill that role. By "fulfill," I mean graciously

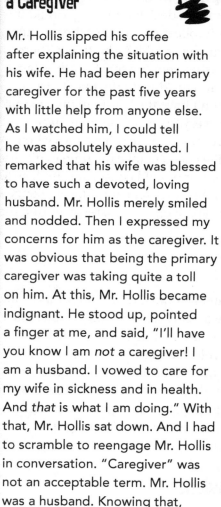

I'm *Not* a Caregiver

Mr. Hollis sipped his coffee after explaining the situation with his wife. He had been her primary caregiver for the past five years with little help from anyone else. As I watched him, I could tell he was absolutely exhausted. I remarked that his wife was blessed to have such a devoted, loving husband. Mr. Hollis merely smiled and nodded. Then I expressed my concerns for him as the caregiver. It was obvious that being the primary caregiver was taking quite a toll on him. At this, Mr. Hollis became indignant. He stood up, pointed a finger at me, and said, "I'll have you know I am *not* a caregiver! I am a husband. I vowed to care for my wife in sickness and in health. And *that* is what I am doing." With that, Mr. Hollis sat down. And I had to scramble to reengage Mr. Hollis in conversation. "Caregiver" was not an acceptable term. Mr. Hollis was a husband. Knowing that, we continued our conversation speaking the same language.

Example

receive the assistance offered. Gracious acceptance is a challenge for many of us!

It is interesting to realize that human beings are born as natural care receivers. Think about it? As a baby, did you resist bottles, clean diapers, shelter, and the loving arms of your parents? Did you resist the assistance needed and wanted as a child? Nope! Babies are naturally gracious care receivers. And, to be honest, that is the *only* time in my life that I have been gracious in receiving. As I matured, I learned by watching my mom that it is better to give than to receive. That lesson was reinforced by the praise and thanks offered each time I offered care to someone. We are taught the preferred role is that of care*giver*. So, when age and illness diminish our capacity to give care and necessitate the acceptance of care, we chafe against the role reversal. We don't want the secondary role. Hence, we struggle to remember how to be gracious care receivers.

Several years ago, I learned of a book that explained the essential nature of caregiving. *A Shepherd Looks at Psalm 23* (1979) by Phillip Keller is a gem of a book. If you are interested in theology, the book does a lovely job of providing insights into Psalm 23. More importantly for the purposes of our discussion, Keller describes the essential nature of the caregiving relationship. As a shepherd, Keller understands what it means to care for his flock. He also understands what it means to be cared for *by* his flock! As described, the relationship between shepherd and sheep is one of *interdependence*. A mutually beneficial relationship. Both parties—shepherd and sheep—have important roles in the relationship. Both parties are dependent on the other for care. Both parties have something of significance to offer. And both parties ultimately benefit from the relationship.

I knew very little about sheep before reading Keller's book. Being from West Texas where cattle rule, I have to admit my opinion of sheep was not favorable. Not the smartest creatures on the planet! But, after reading Keller's book, I realized sheep have something of great importance to teach me. Sheep know how to graciously receive care. They are good at it! Sheep understand that shepherding involves an exchange of gifts between shepherd and sheep. The shepherd (caregiver) provides all aspects of care for the flock: food, water, shelter, protection, medicine, and companionship. In return, the flock (care receiver) sustains the life of the shepherd by providing food, clothing, livelihood, sense of purpose, and companionship. Because of the exchange—the interdependence—shepherd and sheep contribute to and benefit from the process of shepherding (caregiving). Different roles. Equal stature.

The next time you're reluctant to ask for or receive help, take time to thoughtfully reflect on the source of your resistance. Whether a caregiver or care receiver, you may have an occasion when you bristle at the thought of someone else stepping in, taking over, or taking control. In that moment, reflect on WWSD—what would sheep do? Perhaps *ewe* will then know what to do! Sorry, I wanted to *ram* home one last point!

To Summarize...

🔔 Caregiving is not a short-term proposition. So it's very likely that you'll need help along the way from family, friends, and professionals. There are a number of options for sharing the responsibilities of care. However, one size does *not* fit all. Select the model of care that suits the needs, the wants, and the desires of your family. A model may look good on paper. But if it doesn't work well in the trenches, it's of little value.

🔔 In the United States, most people find it difficult to ask for and receive help. We are raised to be independent and self-reliant. Additionally, there may be cultural and family norms that inhibit our ability to ask for help. It's important to identify the sources of our resistance if we are to access the assistance we need and want as caregivers and care receivers.

🔔 Men and women engage the role of caregiver in different ways. It is important to understand how men and women view the role of caregiver so that appropriate and necessary support can be offered.

🔔 We all need role models in life. If you need a role model on how to be a care receiver, look to our good friend the sheep! *Ewe* can't do better than that!

Chapter 17

Tipping Points

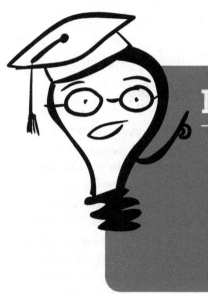

In This Chapter...

- What is a caregiving tipping point?
- Why is guilt so common among caregivers?
- How can families effectively deal with caregiving dilemmas?
- How does the collaborative decision-making process work?

Listening to the stories of countless caregivers over the years, I recognize that families often require an incentive, a motivating factor, before seeking needed assistance with care. In every caregiving story, there is a moment when everything changes. This *tipping point* signifies a change that precipitates a caregiving crisis. The status quo is no longer sufficient to meet the needs of the care receiver. Thus, the plan of care must be revised. A tipping point denotes a game-changing development of concern to one and all.

What does a tipping point look like? There are a variety of situations that prove to be tipping points for families. It just depends on the specifics of the family system and the caregiving concern. However, there are some common occurrences and aspects of aging and illness that serve to precipitate significant, disturbing changes for families. We'll review the more common caregiving tipping points.

Tipping points often spark caregiving dilemmas, a tremendous challenge for families. A *dilemma*, by definition, means that a difficult choice must be made between two equally unappealing alternatives. How a family deals with the dilemma has far-reaching implications for all involved. Using the collaborative decision-making process, families can reach a consensus as to what must be done while avoiding destructive, emotionally charged arguments.

Tipping Point

The point after which everything changes. A caregiving tipping point is often the unwelcome wake-up call that requires families to respond to changing physical, cognitive, or psychosocial conditions. Caregiving tipping points often motivate families to seek additional assistance with caregiving needs as well.

Definition

Living on the Edge

The caregiving journey is a continuous process of change and subsequent transitions. Hence, families are constantly coping and adapting to the changing needs of the care receiver. An approach that worked well in the initial stages of an illness may prove to be inadequate as the illness progresses. However, before a family opts to change the status quo, something significant must occur. A tipping point must be encountered.

As we know, a tipping point is the critical point in a process after which everything changes. It's often the moment when a family realizes the challenge of caring for a loved one is beyond the capacity of the family system. Additional help is needed. Something must change. This realization can be heartbreaking for a family, resulting in tremendous grief and guilt. The situation requires that a decision be made; however, there are no good options. Caregiving dilemmas often generate tremendous stress and conflict within families. Thus, after discussing tipping points, I'll review some ideas on how families can effectively deal with caregiving dilemmas.

Caregiving Tipping Points

What constitutes a caregiving tipping point? Well, it depends. It depends on the specifics of the caregiving situation and the family system. What is a tipping point for one family is an easily absorbed transition for another. However, the more common caregiving tipping points are worthy of reflection if for no other reason than to alert you to the destabilizing influence these situations can have on families. An enhanced awareness of the more common tipping points serves to reinforce our proactive approach to caregiving, right? So let's consider the following caregiving tipping points and the game-changing implications of each.

Acute Medical Incident

Acute medical emergencies are tipping points that throw a family into crisis mode. Heart attack. Stroke. Broken hip. The family reacts to the acute situation, meeting the immediate needs of the care receiver. Gradually, the family assesses the longer-term caregiving needs and identifies the assistance available and required. Depending on the prognosis, the family determines the model of care needed to address the caregiving requirements.

Diagnosis of Serious, Acute Illness or Injury

For acute illnesses and injuries with favorable prognoses, families may be initially stressed trying to meet the short-term caregiving challenges. However, the expectation is that the care receiver and the family will return to "normal" in a relatively short period of time. Hence, the tipping point prompts a short-term aberration, not a life-changing event.

Diagnosis of Chronic/Progressive/Terminal Illness

With the diagnosis of a chronic and/or progressive illness, the family experiences the tipping point differently. The initial shock of the diagnosis is a mental tipping point. The family thinks about life differently. There is a need to plan differently. So families may not have an immediate need for additional assistance, but they know they will at some point. With chronic/progressive/terminal illness, families will experience multiple tipping points as the illness progresses. The intervening times, or plateaus, allow the family to regain a sense of stability before the next tipping point destabilizes the process once again. With each tipping point, families reassess the need for assistance as caregiving needs increase.

Incontinence

Urinary and/or fecal incontinence is a common tipping point for families caring for loved ones at home. Primary caregivers may feel incapable of dealing with this aspect of care. Or, based on the relationship between the caregiver and care receiver, incontinence care is not appropriate. The family must then decide how to respond to this complicating factor. Three possible solutions are the use of incontinence garments and pads for the bed, professional care in the home, or transition to a long-term care community.

Wandering

Many people diagnosed with a progressive dementia, such as Alzheimer's disease, exhibit a behavior known as wandering. This behavior often signifies a tipping point for families caring at home for loved ones with dementia. A person who wanders may leave the house to run a routine errand. Once away from the house, the person becomes disoriented and cannot discern how to return home. This is obviously a very dangerous situation and especially problematic if the primary caregiver works outside the home. The wandering tipping point forces a family to consider additional help at home or the possibility of transition to a memory-specific care community.

Violent and Abusive Behaviors

A tipping point in caregiving often arises when the safety of the caregiver comes into question. For the purposes of our discussion, I'm focusing on violent and abusive behaviors resulting from specific disease processes. We touched on the serious issue of elder abuse and violent care receivers previously. But in the case of progressive neurological conditions, people can become violent and abusive as a consequence of the illness. Compromised caregiver safety is a serious tipping point that prompts family discussions on how to mitigate the threat. Violent and abusive care receivers are difficult to place in long-term care communities. Hence, families oftentimes face limited options and heartbreaking decisions.

May I Walk with You?

Every day, Louise hooked up her two dogs and went for a walk in the neighborhood. It was one of her favorite things to do. Granted, she didn't always remember where she had gone the day before. Such is the life for someone with Alzheimer's disease. But today, she was eager to get outside and walk with her dogs. And she was eager to see Pat.

Pat was a neighbor who lived a few doors down. Interestingly enough, Pat was always outside when Louise walked the dogs. At least the days Louise could remember. Each time, Pat seemed excited to see her and asked, "May I walk with you?" And each time, Louise welcomed the company. She had to admit, there were some days she wasn't exactly sure how to get back home. But Pat knew. So instead of worrying about how to get back home, Louise enjoyed the walk, her dogs, and her new friend.

Louise never knew that her daughter had asked all the neighbors for help. Since the day Louise had trouble returning from the grocery store, her daughter worried about her safety. But she also wanted Louise to be at home for as long as possible. Even though Louise's daughter now lived with her, she worked during the day. So the neighbors were an integral part of the plan to keep Louise safe.

When Pat heard about the daughter's concern, she offered to "watch out" for Louise every morning. More often than not, that was when Louise walked the dogs. Pat said she wouldn't make a big deal about it. She would merely ask Louise if she could join in the walk. Then she would make sure Louise arrived safely back home. As it turned out, Pat thoroughly enjoyed her time with Louise. Now, at the conclusion of every walk, Pat and Louise enjoyed a cup of coffee and cookies. Pat felt good about helping Louise and her daughter. She also felt blessed to be part of Louise's journey. She knew this would be a long and challenging path for Louise and her family. She couldn't change the reality of Alzheimer's disease. But there was one thing Pat could do. She could walk Louise home.

Safety Issues

Concern for the safety of the care receiver is an obvious tipping point in the journey of caregiving. The residence of a care receiver may pose a serious threat if the person is physically and/or cognitively impaired. Or there may be concerns that the primary caregiver is unable to provide adequate care. Whatever the specifics might be, the care receiver is at risk in the current situation. Additional assistance may mitigate the risk in the current environment. If not, transition to a safer location will be required. To knowingly ignore the safety concerns and/or to inadequately meet the needs of a senior in your care are forms of elder abuse called elder neglect. Please know, there are legal implications for inaction and neglect. Do not ignore this tipping point.

Proximity to Family Caregivers

In **Chapter 6**, we explored the issue of long-distance caregiving. It is financially and physically draining for caregivers to travel back and forth in an attempt to care for an aging or ill family member. Additionally, we noted how long-distance caregiving strains intimate as well as business relationships. Consequently, the long-distance caregivers often reach a tipping point when they say enough! At that point, the debate ensues as to whether relocation of the care receiver is the best option. An exploration of local resources (personal and professional) is advisable, as relocation often precipitates the physical and/or cognitive demise of the care receiver.

When Aging in Place Is Not Advisable

In **Chapter 8**, we discussed the concept of aging in place. Basically, it means that you get older where you stand. There is no inference as to the quality of your existence. If we have not done a good job of anticipating and planning for compromised health as we age, we find ourselves in situations that do not accommodate physical or cognitive impairments. When that happens, a tipping point arises that threatens our autonomy and independence. We may be forced to leave our beloved home and transition to a location where additional assistance and care is available. This can be devastating for the entire family.

Roaming Around the Ranch

Standing on the porch, he could see the familiar profile of his father in the corral. His father was conducting the traditional evening ritual of saying good night to the horses. As he watched, Jason longed to remember every detail of the scene. He knew he would need this memory in the days and weeks to come. Jason would need something familiar to support and sustain him after moving his father from the land that he loved. Moving his father into town was the hardest thing Jason would ever do in this lifetime. But there were no other options. Although he and his family loved the remote location of their ranch, the isolation now prohibited his father from living at home.

Jason's father had been diagnosed with Parkinson's disease five years ago. The physical aspects of the illness were challenging enough. But the cognitive impairment proved to be the tipping point. This past winter, Jason spent a frigid, frantic night looking for his father on the ranch. Jason had been out feeding the cows. Upon returning to the house, he realized his father was gone. Jason checked the barn and discovered one of the horses missing as well. Trusting his instincts, Jason saddled up and rode to the most likely place his father would go. He went to the family homestead where his father was born and raised. His father might not remember everything present day, but Jason prayed he would never forget his roots. He prayed his father would always be able to find his way home. Jason's prayers were answered that night.

Jason knew he was lucky that night when he found his father curled up on the porch of his childhood home. The next time, he might not be as fortunate. So he made the gut-wrenching decision to move his father to a care community in town.

As his father concluded the horse ritual, Jason realized this was the last time he would witness his father "at home." Tomorrow, they would make the long drive into town. Jason would do what needed to be done. Then he would make the long drive back to the ranch. Tomorrow night, both he and his father would be in a strange place. His father in town. Jason, alone, at the ranch. Without his father roaming around the ranch, Jason would never again truly feel "at home."

Financial Issues

Illness and the complications associated with aging are costly. Quite often, the care receiver relies on family members to pay for associated costs of care and quite possibly daily living expenses. The financial burden of care often serves as a tipping point requiring modifications to the plan of care or even changes in residence. If the care receiver can no longer afford to pay for housing, the family often provides room, board, and care. This is not a decision to be made lightly or quickly. Family systems work to maintain a tenuous balance during the good times. The introduction of a new member to the household throws the system out of balance on all levels. Although a viable and often-available option, other options should be considered as well.

Domestic Partner Predeceases Care Receiver

When a person's domestic partner dies, it often becomes apparent that the surviving spouse/partner is incapable of living alone. Tipping point! This happens quite often with elderly couples. The surviving spouse/partner keeps it together until the other person dies. Shortly thereafter, the family recognizes the compromised capacity of the surviving spouse/partner. There is already so much change, loss, and grief moving through the family system following the death of a loved one, families should be judicious about any additional change. Consider a less disruptive short-term fix that allows the grieving spouse/partner some time to adjust. Then consider a longer-term solution that may entail the transition to a new place of residence.

Caregiver Guilt

Immediately following the diagnosis of a serious illness, families often make promises that ultimately cannot be honored. A wife promises to never transition her husband to a memory care community. A family commits to keeping their mother at home while handling the demands of ALS (Lou Gehrig's disease). A husband vows to keep his wife at home no matter what. We make these promises with the best of intentions. We intend to honor our commitments. And then something happens. A tipping point. Safety becomes an issue. Another medical condition complicates care. The level of care is beyond our capacity and capabilities. The duration of care exceeds

I Promise

As the doctor explained the situation to Laura, she struggled to understand what had happened over the past forty-eight hours. Just two days ago, she and her husband were doing just *fine*. Well, not totally fine, but they were getting along. The recent complications associated with Charles' diabetes made every day difficult for both of them. But Laura had no qualms about caring for her husband. It's what she wanted to do. It's what she promised to do! However, today the doctor told her that Charles wouldn't be going home. He *couldn't* go home. She would have to make other arrangements for his care by week's end.

Laura failed to hear the rest of the directives recited by the doctor. Instead, she tried to imagine telling her husband of sixty years that he was not going home. Of all the vows she had made in her life, this was the most sacred. She promised to always care for Charles—in their home. Today, a doctor she had only just met informed her that she *had* to break that vow. She no longer heard anything the doctor was saying. The echo of her long-ago vow to care muted all other sounds—"I promise, Charles. Believe me, I promise." Sadly, there are some promises we cannot keep.

IMPORTANT!

expectations. The primary caregiver becomes ill. Unanticipated symptoms complicate care. Regardless of the specifics, we reach a tipping point. From that point forward, everything changes. It's a game changer. Tipping points can also be promise breakers, causing families to feel tremendously guilty.

Guilt is a serious issue for many caregivers. It is an emotion derived from the belief that we have violated personal values and moral standards. Due to circumstances, we cannot honor a previous commitment. This is a heavy burden to bear in addition to the typical stresses of caregiving.

In some instances, primary caregivers resist making difficult decisions because of promises made. This can delay needed care and compromise the safety of both caregiver and care receiver. Sometimes the caregiver needs permission from other family members or health care professionals to make the tough decisions. We need the reassurance that we are doing the best thing for our loved ones. It may not feel right, but it's the best thing, considering the circumstances.

Caregiving Dilemmas

Tipping points commonly precipitate caregiving dilemmas. A *dilemma* is a situation that requires a difficult choice be made between alternatives, neither of which is particularly appealing. Being on the horns of a dilemma is like trying to pick between the lesser of two evils. How do you do that? For example, the various amenities of different long-term care communities matter not when your mother wants to remain in her home. Yet a transition is mandated by circumstances. Not a pleasant situation, to say the very least!

Additionally, tipping points spawn a surge of emotions when families realize they have passed a point of no return. Sorrow. Grief. Sadness. Anger. Disbelief. Guilt. Denial. Frustration. In an already-difficult situation, our emotions can cloud our judgment, increase anxiety, and ignite family arguments.

How can families effectively discuss the options for care? What approach serves to encourage collaboration and productive debate? Well, there are two vital elements when dealing with dilemmas: attitude and process.

The effective and compassionate resolution of caregiving dilemmas hinges on the attitudes of all involved. Although everyone has an opinion about what *should* happen, we need to focus on the greater good. So leave your agenda and ego at the door. This is not about winning an argument. Instead, it's about working together to resolve a very difficult situation.

Even with the best of intentions, families can still be derailed by tipping points. It's not enough to *want* to work together; we need to know *how* to work together. So a process designed to encourage collaboration is quite helpful. Collaborative decision making is a process that assists families struggling with caregiving dilemmas. The process is designed to:

- seek agreement;
- be collaborative;
- encourage cooperation;
- honor all participants;
- include all stakeholders;
- invite participation in the process.

Families can reach consensus by utilizing the collaborative decision-making process. By consensus, I mean an agreement that is supported by the family as a whole. Consensus doesn't mean everyone gets everything they want. However, all family members will be supportive of the ultimate decision. Everyone consents to the decision.

Sounds fabulous, right? So *how* does this happen? How does a family implement the collaborative decision-making process? Consider the following plan of implementation:

Thoughtfully schedule a family meeting. Consider the who, what, when, where, why, and how of the gathering. For those family members geographically dispersed, consider technological options of attendance, such as conference call, Skype, or videoconferencing. Be very sensitive as to where the meeting is held. It is best to pick neutral ground so that no one has home-field advantage. Libraries, offices, restaurants, faith community meeting rooms, or coffee shops offer meeting space worthy of consideration.

Consensus

A general agreement or decision achieved by a group of people. Consensus is not indicative of unanimity. However, it does indicate that all persons in the group consent to support the decision.

Definition

Select meeting facilitator. A nonfamily facilitator is very beneficial if families are highly emotional, argumentative, or confrontational. A nonanxious presence at the meeting serves to control the crowd and to maintain focus on the task at hand.

Establish ground rules for discussion. It is important to establish ground rules for the meeting. People should be reminded that respectful dialogue is the expectation and requirement for participation. Additionally, in the spirit of collaboration, the goal is not to *win* the debate. Rather, the goal is to reach consensus. Acknowledge the difficulty of the situation. Encourage participation. Review the agenda for the meeting.

- Identify the ultimate goal. Succinctly describe the task at hand, the caregiving dilemma that prompted the family meeting.

- Discuss the dilemma. Encourage a respectful discussion of the facts related to the situation. Address concerns or questions. Realize when there are no "good" available options, family members can and will become emotional, frustrated, and angry. Stay focused on the issue. Otherwise, the conversation can devolve into personal attacks and destructive arguments.

- Identify possible options. Identify and debate the available options. Encourage exploration and discussion of the pros and cons related to each option.

- Allow people to emote. Provide people the opportunity to express how they feel about the situation. What's the bottom line for each person? What is acceptable and what is not?

- Listen respectfully. In the spirit of collaboration, everyone needs to be heard. Listening is a critically important aspect of the collaboration process. We need not be in agreement in order to listen respectfully.

- Reach consensus. Consensus is a resolution with broad-based support. It may not be the preference of every family member. However, as a group, every person consents to support the decision.

Tipping points generate tremendous anxiety and stress within family systems. The collaborative decision-making process assists in the resolution of caregiving dilemmas. A good thing indeed!

To Summarize...

- Caregiving tipping points signify changes that often precipitate caregiving crises for families. For whatever reason, the caregiving game changes and there is no going back.

- Caregiving tipping points come in all shapes and sizes. What constitutes a tipping point depends on the care receiver, the family, and specific circumstances. However, there are some common occurrences that typically force families to adjust the plan of care and seek additional assistance.

- Quite often when a tipping point forces a change of plans, previous promises made to the care receiver cannot be kept. The primary caregiver and family subsequently experience a tremendous amount of guilt.

- Caregiving dilemmas are challenging for families. Often, difficult situations arise necessitating difficult decisions after encountering a caregiving tipping point. There are no "good" options or alternatives. So families must choose the lesser of two evils. A collaborative approach to decision making serves to facilitate the process and helps families avoid divisive arguments.

Chapter 18

Flying in Formation: Collaborative Care Takes Flight

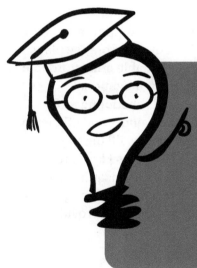

In This Chapter...

- What can geese teach us about caregiving?
- What are the potential benefits of flying in formation?
- How does collaborative care take flight?
- What are the cardinal rules of collaborative care?

Collaborative care is a philosophy of caregiving that encourages the participation of all those affected by a caregiving situation. In the previous chapter, we examined the process and the benefits of collaborative decision making. Once a consensus is reached, how do we then launch and sustain our plans? Every family is unique. Every situation different. So each flight plan will reflect the peculiarities and preferences of those involved. But instead of "winging it," I suggest we look to the skies and observe how geese fly. Geese understand collaborative care!

Collaboration is a way of working together to complete a task or to achieve a common goal. Although collaborative efforts entail the sharing of resources and responsibilities, the process benefits from a point of leadership. In regard to caregiving, the point of leadership is typically the primary caregiver. Even in situations where numerous people share the responsibilities of care, there is typically a primary caregiver coordinating and overseeing the consensus plan of care. However, there is the possibility, and perhaps the need, for shared leadership when coordinating the efforts of numerous caregivers. Each family determines how best to leverage the collective gifts of those involved and thus maximize the benefits of collaborative care.

Technology serves to support and sustain the flight of collaborative plans of care. Readily available and affordable communication, organizational, informational, and scheduling tools enhance the effectiveness and efficiency of collaborative efforts. I'll highlight specific online resources I know to be of benefit to families, organizations (faith communities, disease-specific agencies, etc.), and professional care providers.

Collaboration

An act of working together to achieve a common goal or to complete a task. Participants work interdependently for the mutual benefit of all involved. Collaboration typically requires a leader to coordinate and to oversee the collaborative effort. In the context of caregiving, primary caregivers often provide the necessary leadership.

Definition

The Collaborative Approach to Care

Collaborative care is not a specific, structured model of caregiving; rather, it's a philosophy of caregiving. It's an invitation for all interested parties to actively participate in the caregiving journey. Interdependence is the key to collaborative care and mutually beneficial relationships. I lean on you. You lean on me. Collaboration is defined as two or more people working together to achieve a common goal, committed to the task at hand. Thus, a collaborative process entails the sharing of ideas, perspectives, and knowledge in order to build consensus. Because of this sharing, the strengths of all participants can be leveraged, thereby enriching and improving the overall process.

So think of it this way. Collaborative care promotes the exchange of gifts between the various participants. In instances where there is simply a primary caregiver, collaborative care can be practiced by the caregiving duo. For families choosing to share the responsibilities of care, collaborative care facilitates the allocation of resources and the assignment of tasks. If professional caregivers are part of the plan of care, they can and should be included in the collaborative approach to care. Online resources (discussed later in the chapter) are available to schedule and organize the collaborative efforts of family, friends, and professionals. Basically, the philosophy of collaborative care is applicable to any model or style of caregiving. Working together to achieve common goals facilitates the journey for all involved.

Look to the Skies

Every fall in West Texas, I enjoyed watching geese fly overhead as I worked in the yard with my mom. When we heard the characteristic honking from overhead, we would put down our rakes and take time to witness the migration of geese. We so enjoyed watching the undulating Vs of countless geese against the cobalt blue skies. Glorious! At that time, I didn't appreciate the efficiency of flight or the benefits of flying in formation. However, decades later, I learned how wise our feathered friends truly are.

Several years ago, I attended a retreat in which the image of geese in flight inspired an attitude of cooperation and community. Over the course of the weekend, the facilitators of the event described how and why geese fly in formation. For those of you having a lowly opinion of geese, please reconsider! Geese have much to teach us about community, leadership, and collaboration. Since that retreat, I've noticed organizations using the metaphor of geese in flight to motivate employees. I'm sure you've seen posters of geese in flight with an inspirational quote about teamwork. Or perhaps you've watched the videos on YouTube of geese flying as *The Goose Story* is read (Dr. Harry Clarke Noyes, 1992). Amazing, isn't it? A bird that was once thought to be a bit dense is now an inspiration for corporate development in America!

Collaborative Care

Collaborative care is not a specific, structured model of caregiving; rather, it's a philosophy of caregiving. It's an invitation for all interested parties to actively participate in the caregiving journey. Interdependence, mutually beneficial relationships, is the key to collaborative care.

Perspiration

Do geese have a message for caregivers as well? Absolutely! Geese embody the collaborative approach that is so needed throughout the caregiving journey. Geese work together to achieve common goals and complete identified tasks. Whether a primary caregiver flying solo or a collective of caregivers, we can benefit from the wisdom of geese. So let's explore what can be learned by looking to the skies and observing geese in flight.

Shared Leadership

If you've ever watched geese fly, you've probably noticed that from time to time, the goose at the front of the V drops back in formation. As the lead goose relinquishes the point position, another goose assumes the leadership role. Hence, the entire flock shares in the responsibilities of leadership. This requires inherent trust between all members of the flock. It also requires the willingness of all members to share the leadership role.

What are the potential benefits of shared leadership within the context of caregiving?

- Primary caregivers need not be on "point" all the time. Rotation of leadership provides the necessary breaks to recharge and refresh. Respite occurs routinely as the role of leadership rotates.

- If something were to happen to the primary caregiver, shared leadership ensures that other people are prepared and able to assume the leadership role. There is a Plan B in place for any unexpected events.

- Shared leadership leverages the strengths and abilities of all involved.

- If your family has historically resisted the collaborative approach to care, you might consider initiating a new family legacy of care.

Share the Point Position

Primary caregivers need to look to the skies from time to time for an important life-giving reminder. The point position is not a lifetime assignment. Just like geese, we need to fall back in formation and ride on the tail feathers of others from time to time.

IMPORTANT!

What worked well in the past may not be appropriate today for your current situation. In the case of chronic and progressive illness, shared leadership is a beneficial and effective approach for long-term caregiving.

Fly Faster, Farther

Based on the scientific study of geese in flight, it's been determined that geese in formation fly 71 percent farther than if flying alone. Each goose benefits from the lift generated by other members of the V. Hence, geese fly faster and farther because of the interdependent nature of their relationships. As a goose benefits from the lift generated by the goose in front, that goose in turn generates a beneficial lift for the goose behind. The lead goose expends the greatest energy since there is no beneficial lift at the point position. As noted above, that is why shared leadership is so important. As the lead goose tires, the rotation of leadership provides a much-needed break to rest and recover. Consequently, the flock flies faster and farther in formation.

How does "uplift" translate to the journey of caregiving?

- The average duration of the caregiving journey is 4.6 years. With the anticipated increased incidence of Alzheimer's disease over the next thirty years, the caregiving journey will become even longer. Hence, caregivers flying in formation will be better able to manage long-term caregiving. The ability to "fly farther" will become increasingly important in the coming years.

- "Flying in formation" generates a sense of community predicated on interdependence. Each person contributes to and benefits from the collective efforts of everyone involved. Caregivers feel supported and "uplifted" by a sustaining community.

Collaborative care, flying in formation, helps maintain the health and well-being of the primary caregiver. Collaborating with other people reduces the "drag" on the primary caregiver and thus reduces stress. As noted previously, chronic stress compromises the immune system, making caregivers more susceptible to illness. Riding on the "lift" of others mitigates this risk.

Life Doesn't Have to Be a Drag

If you are weary of flying solo as a primary caregiver, get back in formation! It can be an uplifting experience to share the journey of caregiving with supportive family and friends.

Pure Genius!

Stay in Formation

Geese are just like people in some ways. Geese don't always do the wisest things. Watching geese in flight, you'll occasionally see a goose break from formation. However, it is not long before the rogue goose wings its way back to the flock. Error recognized and rectified. A goose immediately feels the drag of flying solo. Working harder to fly, the goose becomes fatigued.

As caregivers, we experience the same thing. For whatever reason, we break formation with our collaborators of care. Usually, in short order, we realize that flying solo is a tough proposition indeed. We feel the drag. However, unlike our friend the goose, human beings take a little longer to admit the error of our ways. In fact, some caregivers wait until the wings fall off before honking for help! Word to the wise—stay in formation.

In-Flight Cheerleaders

Have you ever noticed that geese are a raucous bunch? When geese fly, they honk incessantly! What is that? Although the honking may serve to annoy you at some level, honking motivates and encourages geese to fly. It's like flying with a flock of feathered cheerleaders. Keep going! Keep flapping! You can do it!

As caregivers, we often need encouragement as well. That is one of the reasons a collaborative approach to care is so incredibly important. If we become isolated, there is no one to "honk" when we feel discouraged and exhausted. So stay in formation. Surround yourself with people who honk when you need it most. Believe me, honking is a blessing to weary caregivers. So don't be shy. Honk with gusto!

Complete the Flight

Geese exhibit a profound commitment to each other. Geese companion each other to the end of the flight. Scientists observe that when a goose falls out of formation due to injury or illness, at least one other goose breaks rank as well. The impaired goose will be companioned to recovery or to death. Either way, the goose will not be alone. This commitment to companioning is an essential aspect of collaborative care. Committing to care for someone is a moral obligation. We commit to companion that person to the end of their flight. It is not always an easy journey; however, we are called to courageously witness the completion of the flight.

How to Fly in Formation

In order to fly in formation, you need a flight plan. Whether you have two people or one hundred people involved in your collaborative plan of care, the caregiving process is facilitated greatly by a little organization. Technology serves to streamline the organizational aspects of care. Online resources have proven to be blessings for those coordinating the collective efforts of family and friends.

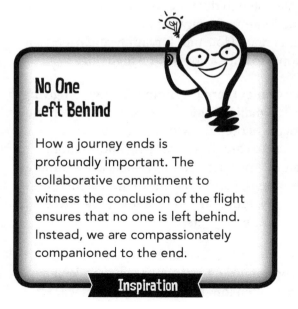

No One Left Behind

How a journey ends is profoundly important. The collaborative commitment to witness the conclusion of the flight ensures that no one is left behind. Instead, we are compassionately companioned to the end.

Inspiration

🔍 Lotsa Helping Hands (lotsahelpinghands.com): From personal and professional experience, I have witnessed the benefits of this free online resource. Families create password-protected websites to streamline scheduling of caregiving tasks, communicate with participants, post information, and access information. You don't have to be a

Stay in Touch

We know that caregiving can be stressful and isolating for the caregiver and care receiver. So it's important to stay in touch with family and friends throughout the journey. I recently participated in a CaringBridge community created for a colleague of mine. Over the course of two years, friends and family members posted over fifty thousand messages. Talk about staying in touch!

Inspiration

computer wizard to utilize this site. The process is very intuitive, and the website has good technical support for any question that might arise. Lotsa Helping Hands is a fabulous resource for short-term or long-term caregiving needs. The site serves to organize, to connect, and to benefit the caregiving journey. Check it out. You'll have a flight plan in place before you know it!

🔍 CaringBridge (caringbridge.org): CaringBridge is a free online option worthy of consideration. The site offers communication and organizational tools for families dealing with short-term or long-term caregiving issues. The site was originally established to facilitate the conveyance of information about the status of care receivers. This is one of the best sites if you're interested in documenting the "conversation" between family and friends. I know of many families that, after the fact, printed off the postings and created journals for family and friends. It is often comforting for people to have a copy of the flight log.

🔍 AARP Caregiving Resource Center (aarp.org/home-family/caregiving): This is a treasure chest of information for caregivers. There are online tools that facilitate the process of preparing to care. Links to caregiving blogs. Recent news of interest to caregivers. Housing information. Videos. Insurance calculators. And so much more! Take a few minutes to explore the available resources. I am sure you will find something of benefit for you and your family. From takeoff to landing, the AARP site serves as a valuable resource for caregivers.

🔍 Skype (skype.com): Skype is an online service that allows people to communicate by voice, by video, and by instant message. When organizing caregiving efforts, often long-distance caregivers want to be involved. If unable to be physically present, Skype serves to bridge the gap. Conference calls facilitate the needed discussions as well. However, when emotions are raw and families are stressed, the video component of Skype allows us to witness the facial expressions and body language of those involved. Why fly by instruments when you can access a clear line of sight? Seeing is believing.

 Facebook (facebook.com): Depending upon the online habits of those involved, Facebook may or may not be a valuable resource. If those involved in the plan of care check Facebook once in a blue moon, this resource will be of little benefit to the caregiving efforts. However, many Facebook users remain logged into Facebook 24/7 and check the various postings at least thirty times per day! In that case, Facebook serves to connect, organize, and support the collaborative efforts of caregivers. Thus, you need to know the online habits of those involved in the plan of care. Flying in formation is a general approach to caregiving. The navigational instruments you choose to chart the course of care are up to you.

The Cardinal Rules of Collaborative Care

What else do we need to launch a collaborative plan of care? We examined the metaphor of geese flying in formation to guide our approach to collaborative care. We identified beneficial resources and online tools that facilitate the organization and sustainability of collaborative efforts. Seems like we have everything in place for a successful flight. But, as with all flights, we need to do one more thing. We need to run through a preflight checklist to ensure a safe flight. So I invite you to run through the following checklist before launching a plan of care. The preflight checklist doesn't guarantee a smooth flight. But the preflight routine prepares you to handle whatever happens in flight. The cardinal rules of collaborative care help ensure that we are prepared to care.

The cardinal rules of collaborative care encourage caregivers and care receivers to do the following:

 Be honest—caregiving can be stressful and usually is!

 Be aware of your attitudes—attitude is everything.

🔍 Be realistic—no one person must/can do everything.

🔍 Be proactive—anticipate needs and plan ahead.

🔍 Be gentle with yourself and others—caregiving is *not* about perfection.

🔍 Be knowledgeable—gather needed information.

🔍 Be open to new possibilities—allow others to help.

🔍 Be specific and direct—let others know exactly what you need and want.

🔍 Be organized—coordinate care.

Now sit back, relax, and enjoy your flight!

To Summarize...

🔍 Collaborative care is an approach to caregiving that invites people to participate in the process. Interdependent relationships are the foundation of collaborative care. I lean on you. You lean on me. Mutually beneficial.

🔍 Geese serve as a wonderful metaphor for the collaborative approach to care. Because geese fly in formation, they are able to fly 71 percent farther while reducing the stress for all involved. Geese may not be the smartest bird in the sky, but geese certainly have something to teach human beings about caregiving. Flying solo is not always the best flight plan for caregiving.

🔍 Organization facilitates the collaborative approach to care. There are numerous online resources available to family caregivers to launch the initial plan of care and to sustain the ongoing caregiving efforts.

🔍 Before launching a collaborative plan of care, remember the preflight checklist. The cardinal rules of collaborative care prepare us well for the duration of the flight. Review the rules often, and make course corrections as needed in flight.

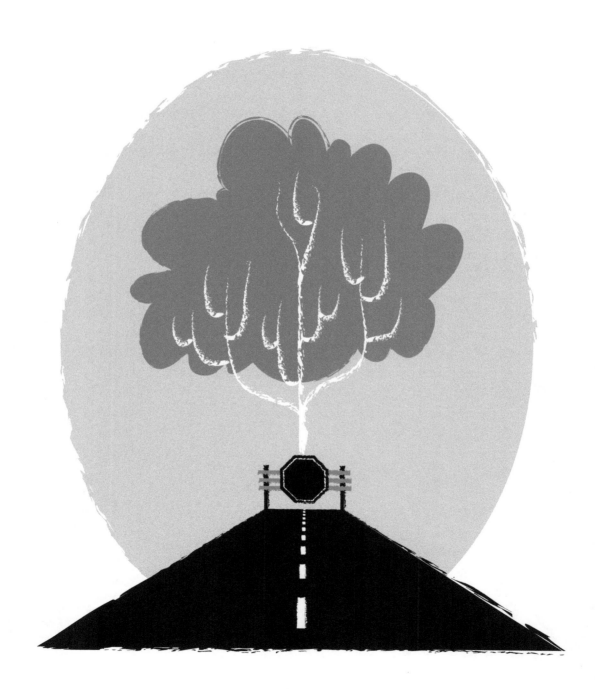

Part 5

The End of the Road

Every journey has an end. Thus, the journey of caregiving will conclude at some point for the caregiver(s) and care receiver. Quite possibly, the ending is cause for celebration due to the full recovery of the care receiver. But not all endings are cause for celebration. With advanced age and terminal illness, the caregiving journey ultimately ends in the death of the care receiver. How we approach the end of the road as caregivers and care receivers is worthy of examination and consideration. We need to prepare well for this part of the journey if we are to be engaged instead of afraid. Yes, there are many changes and losses to be endured along the way. However, have you ever considered what is to be gained as we courageously walk to the end of the road? Sometimes it is in losing that we gain the most.

Chapter 19

Life and Loss

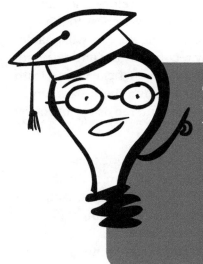

In This Chapter...

- Why is loss an inherent part of life?
- What do we have to lose as caregivers and care receivers?
- What is bereavement overload?
- What do you expect?

Loss. Not a pleasant proposition. However, over the course of a lifetime, we experience a multitude of losses. Caregiving exacerbates the experience of loss due to the compressed timeframe over which loss occurs and the magnitude of losses presented by aging and illness. Losses grab our hearts, cloud our vision, muddy our thoughts, and derail our lives. However, the times of greatest loss often prove to be the opportunities for greatest growth. It's a tough way to evolve, but no one said life was easy. And they were right!

What do we risk losing as we age or as illness compromises our health? It's important to consider and to anticipate the likely losses encountered as a caregiver and care receiver. We can't fully prepare for future losses. However, a realistic assessment of the situation helps prepare for the eventuality.

Many of the physical and cognitive losses will obviously impact the plan of care. But there are other losses oftentimes overlooked that generate a tremendous amount of *grief*. Grief is the natural response to a significant loss. It's a process that involves—often overwhelms—our emotions, thoughts, and behaviors. Grieving is one of the hardest things we do as human beings. Since caregiving includes a myriad of losses, caregivers and care receivers can be consumed by grief. The losses of control, relationships, independence, belonging, and purpose are often unrecognized and therefore discounted. Thus, a heightened awareness to the possible losses along the way will enable us to readily recognize grief and respond in compassionate, beneficial ways. Death is the ultimate loss. But there are many other losses encountered as we journey to the end of the road.

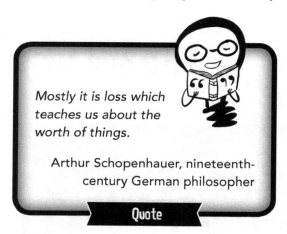

Mostly it is loss which teaches us about the worth of things.

Arthur Schopenhauer, nineteenth-century German philosopher

Quote

Attitude informs and influences the lived experience from start to finish. But attitude is *critically* important when dealing with the challenges and changes posed by aging and illness. When the losses associated with aging and illness begin piling up and grief threatens to consume us, how will we react? Will we choose to be victims of change and loss? Or will we choose to integrate the losses into our lives and grow from the experience? How we choose to engage this part of the journey not only informs our personal experience but also serves as a legacy for our family and friends.

Loss—A Natural Consequence of Life

In **Chapter 3**, we recognized life as a continuous process of change. We know it, but that doesn't mean we like it! We love our routines and the illusion that we are in control. Change highlights the uncertainty of life. If you're like most people, you don't do well with uncertainty or mystery. Instead, we prefer to know what lies ahead and plan accordingly. The other disconcerting aspect about change is the loss necessitated by change. Change, by definition, means that something ends. The ending is followed by a period of adjustment or transition before we reengage with life. It's the endings—the losses—that make the changes experienced as caregivers and care receivers so incredibly poignant. And so we grieve.

Grief is often described as the price we pay for investing ourselves in life. In the midst of profound grief, I have often thought the price too high. In hindsight, I realize my experiences of loss and grief are foundational to who I am, what I do, and who I choose to become. Although I wish there were an easier way to learn transformative life lessons, I am forever grateful for the hard-earned wisdom.

One of the greatest challenges for caregivers and care receivers is the magnitude and volume of change endured as the caregiving journey unfolds. We can experience change fatigue as incremental changes accumulate. We feel overwhelmed by the subsequent losses and grief. We barely have time to feel the grief of one loss before another wave of loss crashes on our shores.

Now rest assured, there are ways to avoid many of the painful losses of life. You can choose to insulate and isolate yourself to the extent there is little risk of attachment. If unattached, you have little exposure to loss and subsequent grief. It's a very safe way to exist. But is it enough to merely exist? Just going through the motions? Personally, I think not. I learned the hard way that playing it safe poses a greater risk than investing fully in life. Limiting the possibility of loss limits your experience of life.

Grief

Grief is the natural response to a significant loss. It is a process involving a variety of emotions, thoughts, and behaviors. Grief is a function of attachment. If we never became involved, invested, or committed to other people, places, or things, there would be no basis for grief because there would be no perceived loss. Our ability and willingness to attach makes us vulnerable to loss and grief.

Definition

Looking at Change and Loss

Our experience of change and loss depends on our perspective. And our perspective depends on our role in the caregiving journey. Caregivers and care receivers are looking at change and loss from different ends of the telescope. What may seem monumental to you may be of little consequence to your

Playing It Safe

The death of my mom had an extraordinary impact on my life. My mom died when I was twenty-four. Being relatively young, I had little experience with death and consequently had no idea how to process her death. I didn't know how to grieve and mourn. I didn't know what to do with my pain and sorrow.

The year following my mom's death brought additional, significant changes that served to distract my attention. It wasn't a conscious choice to ignore my pain, but a pattern of behavior that evolved over time. It wasn't until I experienced another significant loss in life, my divorce, that I realized how my unmourned grief served to hold me back and weigh me down. Unconsciously, I had decided that I would not allow anyone else to get close enough to hurt me again. I would *never* again feel the intensity of pain I felt for my mom. I opted to emotionally disengage from life.

Well, for twelve years, I was quite successful at keeping people at arm's length. I lived a very safe life. No major highs. No major lows. I flatlined. Believe me, it's an incredibly effective way to live if you want to be absolutely numb. But the price for being pain free is that you feel nothing at all. Strangely enough, when the walls came tumbling down in the midst of my divorce, I relished the sense of emotional pain because I felt alive again. I once again felt something!

Reengaging life has been both challenging and invigorating. Being open and vulnerable to the losses of life is certainly difficult at times. And yet, despite the risk of loss, I could never imagine playing it safe again. I don't want to exit this life untarnished and untouched. I hope to exit "gently used," deeply loved, and fully invested in life.

aging father. The impact of the change and subsequent loss depends on the meaning given—the significance and the implications of the loss. If you recall, in **Chapter 9**, we discussed how meaning transforms the experience of suffering. Well, the same is true for change and loss. The meaning attributed to a change is predicated on our unique perspective.

For example, let's say your father falls down the stairs and breaks a hip. The change in his physical stature means something different to your father than it does to you. Your father experiences a loss of independence and autonomy. He may also lose confidence in his ability to live alone. You, on the other hand, perceive the change differently as a child who lives two thousand miles away. You experience the change as the loss of freedom to live your own life. You've lost control! You may also lose the image of your father as the independent patriarch. Same event. Different perspective. Different sense of loss. So the change is understood uniquely by each person who will then have a unique sense of loss as a consequence of the change. This explains why family members react differently to the same event.

Regardless of our role in the caregiving process, we are all at risk of experiencing a variety of changes and losses. In the following section, we will highlight the more common and concerning losses associated with aging and illness.

What Do We Have to Lose?

When presenting programs on grief and loss, I realize most people attend the programs thinking we'll focus exclusively on death losses. However, as you know, we grieve all kinds of losses. Yes, death is the ultimate loss and often the most challenging. But it's important to recognize all losses so that the needed process of grief and mourning ensues. As we will discuss in **Chapter 20**, unmourned losses become impediments in life. The first step is loss recognition. Then we can begin the hard work of integrating loss into our life through the process of grief and mourning. Not an easy task by any means. However, absolutely necessary.

So what changes and subsequent losses can we anticipate as we walk to the end of the road, as a caregiver or care receiver? As you read through the various losses, are there any that make you a bit uneasy? Have you experienced a similar loss in the past? Perhaps anticipating a similar loss in the future? I invite you to take note of the things that make you uncomfortable. Often this uneasiness is indicative of losses that have been ignored or discounted in your past. Consider your discomfort an invitation for reflection. If by chance you discover unmourned grief from past losses, **Chapter 20** explains the grief and mourning process.

Physical Changes and Losses

Physical changes and losses due to aging and illness are often the most obvious. As a natural consequence of aging, we decline physically. Outward signs of age are concerning to most of us. We lament the loss of our youthful appearance. However, we will *not* go gently into that good night! We spend billions of dollars annually on cosmetic fixes to hide the evidence of aging. We also feel the consequences of physical changes as we struggle to get out of bed on cold mornings. We no longer bend and bounce back as we once did as supple teenagers. I can no longer hit a two hundred–yard drive, much to my dismay! And, with enough time, our organs will no longer be capable of performing the necessary bodily functions to sustain life. When injury or illness enters the system, it's as if we put the "pedal to the metal" on the aging process. The normal aging process accelerates, often causing a precipitous decline.

As if the physical changes and losses were not enough, these initial losses precipitate other losses. The proverbial domino effect. If you can no longer climb the stairs leading to your bedroom and master bath, guess what? You may have to move to a more suitable residence. If you are unable to see due to macular degeneration, you will need to surrender your car keys and rely on public transportation or the kindness of friends and family. So be prepared, my friends. Physical changes and losses almost always generate ripples in your pond of tranquility. One loss leads to another. Find the Dramamine if you are prone to motion sickness!

> *Think of life as a terminal illness, because if you do, you will live it with joy and passion, as it ought to be lived.*
>
> Anna Quindlen, American author and journalist, Pulitzer Prize winner, author of *A Short Guide to a Happy Life* (2000)
>
> **Quote**

Cognitive Changes and Losses

As a middle-aged woman, I have moments when I wonder if my wiring is still working! I would imagine you have experienced similar situations as well. You can't remember a name or phone number. Then, thirty minutes later—*voila*! Please know, this is not necessarily indicative of a more serious problem such as dementia. Instead, it is reflective of the natural aging process of human beings. As we age, our brains slow down. The information is still available. Just takes a little longer to access. I liken it to the difference in Internet speeds. When I was thirty, my brain worked as if I was hooked up to high-speed Internet. I could access information instantaneously! Today, I access the Internet using the old dial-up modem. Remember those? We clicked the icon, and our computers made the strangest noises. We had to wait a few minutes (can you imagine?), but the connection was eventually made. The same is true for my brain today. I eventually connect. Just takes a bit more time and patience! Now this may seem like a minor loss. An annoyance and aggravation, for sure. However, for people who know the arduous journey of dementia, this loss of mental acuity is frightening because it is reminiscent of past experiences within the family. So, again, we need to be sensitive as to what the loss means to the person.

In the case of progressive and vascular dementia, the losses associated with cognitive changes are devastating and life changing for all concerned. As we will discuss in **Chapter 20**, the long duration of dementia care is particularly challenging because of the repeated cycle of change, loss, grief, and transition. Change fatigue as well as anticipatory grief magnify the sense of loss.

Loss of Good Health

As we age, there is often a diagnosis or an event that signifies we no longer enjoy good health. The doctor calls with the news that the biopsy was positive. We experience chest pains after climbing a flight of stairs. We're awakened by severe abdominal pain. Whatever the case might be, we now feel a bit more vulnerable regarding our health and well-being. If the change in our health status is significant enough, there will be subsequent changes and losses. How we choose to confront this loss has implications for the quality of life we experience.

That's Life

Carlotta never ceases to amaze me. Over the past twenty years, she's dealt with more medical issues than any one person should have to contend with in a lifetime: heart surgery, diabetes, renal failure, dialysis, retinopathy, and chronic obstructive pulmonary disease. Seems like more than her fair share, to say the least. At dinner one evening, I marveled at her incredibly positive attitude in light of all these medical challenges. She said in her very matter-of-fact manner, "What are you going to do? That's life. You just have to get on with it." And so she does—with a great deal of style and flair!

Pure Genius!

Loss of Youth

Some people seem quite adept at aging gracefully, while others fight the forces of nature with every fiber of their being. Again, how this loss is experienced and mourned depends on the meaning given to the loss. If physical youth is of little importance to you, it will not be a significant loss. I remember as a young child looking at the image of a very old woman in a *National Geographic* magazine. Before I could comment on her grizzled looks and countless wrinkles, my mom shared her impressions. She held the magazine with reverence and touched the picture of the woman gently. Then she looked at me and said, "What an incredibly beautiful woman. I would love to know the story behind each wrinkle." Needless to say, my understanding of age and beauty changed that day. Loss of youth has more to do with attitude than with outward appearance. May we all remain young at heart.

Loss of Relationships

The loss of relationships is one of the most daunting aspects of aging and illness. We know ourselves in relation to other people. When those relationships change or end, our sense of loss is profound. Relationships are lost for a variety of reasons: death, divorce, alienation, dissension, and role changes. We'll discuss death loss extensively in **Chapters 21** and **22**. So keep reading!

In the context of caregiving, relationships may not end, but they certainly change. When we assume the role of caregiver or care receiver, we often neglect our intimate role of wife, husband, daughter, or son. When the demands of caregiving are extreme, it is difficult to find the time to "be" anything other than the caregiver. As a care receiver, our sense of self may be highly distorted, making it difficult to "be" ourselves. This often occurs in the case of role reversals. When an adult child assumes responsibility for the care of an aging parent, the child becomes the parent in the relationship. This is typically a difficult transition for both parties. Sometimes, having the courage to name what is happening opens the door to a beneficial conversation.

Loss of Home—Sense of Belonging

Aging and illness often necessitate a change of residence due to physical, cognitive, or financial changes. The transition causes a tremendous amount of grief associated with the loss of a home. Far too often, this loss is unrecognized and therefore diminished. Before deeming new residents of a long-term care community depressed, perhaps we should take the time to understand the source of the sadness. Yes, they are probably depressed as a natural part of the grieving process. However, that doesn't mean the residents are clinically depressed! They are grieving the loss of a home and a foundational sense of belonging. Antidepressant drugs do nothing to facilitate the grieving process. The drugs merely subdue the emotions and reflect a lack of understanding on the part of health care providers. Often the best medicine we have to offer is our willingness to listen and to be present to the raw grief of another person.

Loss of Faith

If life has not lived up to your expectations, you probably have some burning questions on your lips for whoever or whatever you deem sacred in this life. Aging and illness pose tremendous challenges. Consequently, many of us rely heavily on our foundational beliefs to support and sustain us during the times that try our souls. If we feel abandoned, duped, or betrayed, it often results in a loss of faith. These are the dark nights of the soul that usually require compassionate and knowledgeable companions. Reinforcing a shaky foundation also requires a tremendous amount of courage, commitment, and patience. Rome wasn't built in a day. Reconnecting with our sense of the divine takes time.

Loss of Purpose

Loss of purpose is of concern for both caregivers and care receivers. Care receivers who are compromised physically and/or cognitively may feel as if they have little left to offer the world. And, as we all know, we all need a sense of purpose in life. We need to feel as if we are contributing in meaningful ways. The challenge then becomes recognizing new ways in which meaningful contributions can be made. For caregivers, the loss of purpose often occurs at the conclusion of the caregiving journey. What is the caregiver supposed to do now? For those people who closely identify with the role of caregiver, this is a significant loss and difficult transition.

This Must Be So Hard for You

As I was leaving the assisted living community, I noticed a woman sitting alone in the foyer. There was something about her that compelled me to stop and say hello. When she looked up, I recognized an overwhelming sadness in her eyes. She invited me to sit down, if I had time. Although I had another appointment later in the day, I sensed she needed to talk. She needed someone to listen. So I pulled up a chair and learned of her sorrow.

She explained that she had recently moved and was trying to adjust to her "new home." She had already met some lovely people. Participated in some activities. But it wasn't home. When I asked about her previous home, her eyes filled with tears. She and her husband had shared a home for fifty years. Raised a family. Celebrated holidays. Endured hardships. Created memories. It's where she felt she belonged. As the tears streamed down her face, I said, "This must be so hard for you. I am so sorry for your loss." She seemed a bit startled by my remark. Then, upon reflection, she realized something of great importance. She was grieving. It mattered not how hard she tried to like her new residence. Until she mourned the loss of her previous home, she wouldn't be able to move on.

As I rose to leave, she gave me a big hug and thanked me for our brief conversation. She said, "Thank you for taking the time to listen and to hear my pain."

Loss of Financial Security

Due to the increased costs of care and increased longevity, many people incur extraordinary expenses at the end of life. On top of all the other losses encountered throughout the caregiving journey, the loss of financial security just adds insult to injury. This particular loss has practical implications for the surviving family. If all available financial resources are depleted during the caregiving journey, the survivors may be at risk of losing a great deal more after the death of the care receiver (residence, etc.).

Loss of Control

Progressive illness and aging are two things beyond our control. We certainly can't halt the aging process, nor can we change the nature of an illness. Whether for ourselves or our loved ones, this loss of control infuriates and frustrates us. We feel powerless to influence the process. Vulnerable. Exposed. As we'll discuss in **Chapter 21**, the dying process is one of relinquishing control. For those of us who covet our sense of control, this is an intimidating challenge indeed. Perhaps the invitation for growth is in recognizing what is within our control and what is not.

Loss of Hope

As illness and aging advance, caregivers and care receivers often experience a loss of hope. Hope for cure. Hope for remission. Hope for a longer life. Hope for a future. The loss is felt when the reality of the situation becomes clear. The hope to avoid death is not possible. However, that doesn't necessarily mean there is *no* hope. Is there hope that pain and symptoms can be well managed? Hope to remain at home? Hope to be companioned by family and friends to the end of the road? Regardless of the situation, there is always hope. The challenge is in recognizing that hope evolves as conditions change.

Loss of Independence

In the United States, loss of independence is a pervasive fear. We cherish our ability to self-determine and to captain our own ship. A major symbol of independence is car keys. Being able to drive whenever, wherever, and for whatever reason equates to independence. My heart goes out to anyone who must compel a family member or friend to relinquish the car keys. It is usually not a pleasant encounter! For the entire year following my conversation with Aunt Jane (my godmother), she referred to me as "that woman who *took* the car keys away." More to the point, I was the one who stole her independence. Quite honestly, I don't think Aunt Jane ever forgave me for that transgression!

At the end of life, our ability to make health care decisions may come into question. If we are deemed to be incapable of making our own decisions, we have lost independence. This is when advance directives serve families well. As noted in **Chapter 12**, it's not just the required legal documents that

---

Pure Genius!

Shall We Dance?

It was a tough day for Ben. It was one of those days when he realized he wasn't remembering. Typically, a very difficult time for those diagnosed with dementia. So he was frustrated, angry, scared, and sad. He no longer felt in control of his life.

As we were chatting, I heard music coming from the dining hall. Ben immediately brightened at the sound of music. He asked if I danced. Now, I can do many things well, but dancing is not one of them. Confessing my shortcoming, Ben assured me that he could teach me how to dance. With that, he held out his hand and asked, "Madame, shall we dance?" Well, how could I refuse an invitation like that?

I have to say, I have never danced so well. Ben was masterful and quite patient with me. With Ben in the lead, all I had to do was follow. And I did. He was in control of the dance.

That day, I learned how to waltz. But I learned so much more from Ben. He demonstrated that even when life seems to be out of control, there are opportunities to take the lead. Knowing that, taking the lead in life even for a short time provides the confidence and the desire to persevere.

facilitate the transition of decision making. Rather, it's the conversations between care receiver and family members that establish the foundation of understanding to serve the person well. Loss of independence will remain a fear for most of us. However, with plans in place for a smooth changing of the guards, there is hope that our wishes will be respected and honored.

Loss of Life

Loss of life, the ultimate loss, will be discussed extensively in **Chapter 21**. However, there is one aspect of the death loss I want to highlight now. As caregivers companioning terminal care receivers, we'll experience the pain of saying goodbye to that person. But for the person who is dying, how many goodbyes are needed or wanted? We recognize the surviving family and friends benefit from bereavement support. Yet, perhaps for those who are dying, a little grief counseling would be advisable as well. Think about it. How many people, places, things, and critters will you bid adieu prior to your final departure? This is truly a monumental task worthy of consideration. In **Chapter 21**, we'll delve into the issue of saying goodbye at the end of life.

An Overabundance of Loss

Although the previous list of possible losses is far from comprehensive, it's evident that we'll experience numerous losses as we complete our journey. The losses caused by aging and illness generate a tremendous amount of grief. If change is continuous and precipitous, the grief can become overwhelming for both caregivers and care receivers.

In the 1970s, Robert Kastenbaum coined the term "bereavement overload." As a psychologist and gerontologist, he witnessed the impact that multiple losses or losses in rapid succession had on individuals. This often occurs in tragic events that result in multiple casualties. Bereavement overload is also experienced if our friends and family predecease us in rapid succession.

Bereavement typically refers to the mourning associated with a death loss. So I would suggest modifying Kastenbaum's term to reflect the multiple losses experienced by caregivers and care receivers. *Grief overload* encompasses death losses as well as the many losses discussed previously. The term is actually of little importance. Just be aware that the journey of caregiving poses numerous losses for caregivers and care receivers alike. Hence, we need to be attentive to our need and the need of others to grieve and mourn our losses.

Attitude Makes *All* the Difference

Contemplating the various and sundry losses posed by aging and illness is hard. By now, you may be a bit subdued. You might be rethinking your lifelong travel plans. Is there a way to avoid the end of the road? Thus far, it doesn't sound too appealing. Why in the world would you *choose* a trip that promises a high probability of loss en route with the guaranteed termination point being death? Doesn't sound like the idyllic summer vacation to me!

And yet, isn't this the reality of the back nine holes of life? If you're a golfer, you understand the metaphor. If not, let me explain. A round of golf consists of eighteen holes, a front nine and a back nine. At the conclusion of the front nine, you make "the turn" and tee off on the back nine. I equate the turn with midlife. So, as we tee off on the tenth hole, we know we're on the downhill side of life. We just don't know how fast we will complete the back nine. It could be a leisurely stroll to the clubhouse or an all-out sprint. The goal is to stay in the fairways and avoid all the hazards.

> ### Bereavement Overload
>
> The experience of being overwhelmed by multiple death losses or losses in rapid succession. This could be the result of a tragic incident resulting in numerous casualties. Or, as is often the case for older adults, it is experienced when numerous peers and family members succumb to advanced age and/or illness over a short period of time.
>
> **Definition**

However, realistically, we'll end up in the weeds from time to time, veer into a water hazard, or enjoy some time in the sand. I'm one of those golfers who gets my money's worth. I see the *entire* golf course—fairways, greens, *and* hazards. Such is the nature of life as well.

In life, as in golf, our experience of the round depends on our attitude. If we expect to encounter only fairways and greens for the entire eighteen holes, we will no doubt be aghast and dismayed by the view from the rough. We might panic after losing four or five balls, wondering if we'll be able to complete the round. Or perhaps the round takes a bit longer than we anticipated. As twilight approaches, we fear not being able to see the pin on the eighteenth green. We've come this far. We want to savor that final putt and call it a day. So my question is this. How do you react if your "round" doesn't unfold as planned? What is your attitude when confronted by the hazards and subsequent losses of life? Consider this carefully, because attitude makes *all* the difference.

Happy New Year!

New Year's Eve has never been a major occasion in my life. However, there is one New Year's Eve I will *never* forget. The year I shared New Year's Eve with my best friend, JoAnne, and fifteen women from her volunteer association was stellar!

We gathered at a friend's house to eat dinner and play games until midnight. JoAnne and I, both in our fifties, were the youngsters in the group. Everyone else was over seventy. An amazing gathering of women, to say the very least! Over the course of the evening, these ladies exhibited a profound appreciation of life. Despite, or perhaps because, these ladies had experienced their fair share of losses in life, they knew how to seize the moment and enjoy! Who knew you could have that much fun playing dominos? And it wasn't easy. Half of the ladies were hard of hearing, and half were vision impaired. So JoAnne and I spent most of the night reading the dominos or repeating what was said. What a hoot!

When recalling that New Year's Eve, I marvel at the women in attendance. Each woman had lost so much over the course of a lifetime. Yet they chose not to be defined by loss. They were not victims of life. As I listened to story after story that evening, I heard not one complaint, whine, or moan. Instead, I heard courage, hope, confidence, faith, love, and commitment. These ladies had every reason in the world to despair. Yet they chose to be delightful. Attitude makes *all* the difference!

As we tee it up on the back nine, we're wise to have realistic expectations. We'll experience more loss than we ever imagined. It's the nature of the game. So expect to see more than just fairways and greens! The challenge then becomes how we address life losses when attempting to hack our way out of the rough. In **Chapter 20**, we'll review the basics of grief, mourning, and bereavement. Becoming grief savvy serves us well. We learn how to "come to grips" with our losses.

To Summarize...

Loss is a part of life, a consequence of the ever-changing nature of life. Change, by definition, means that something ends. Endings result in a sense of loss. And the human response to loss is grief. Death is the ultimate loss—and often the most difficult loss. However, to integrate any significant loss into our lives, we must grieve and mourn.

Grief is the natural response to a significant loss. It's a process that involves—often overwhelms—our emotions, thoughts, and behaviors. Grieving is one of the hardest things we do as human beings. Since caregiving includes a myriad of losses, caregivers and care receivers can be consumed by grief.

Within the context of caregiving, we are at risk of losing a myriad of things. Although we can't adequately prepare for all losses, an awareness of and sensitivity to the various losses is beneficial for caregivers and care receivers.

Bereavement overload is the experience of multiple death losses over a very short period of time. Grief overload is a term that includes all types of losses; it is the experience of multiple losses in a compressed time span. The journey of caregiving includes the risk of grief overload for caregivers and care receivers.

What are your expectations for the back nine holes of life? If your expectations are unrealistic, you will be sorely disappointed. The attitude we assume in confronting the hazards of life determines how we will conclude the round.

Chapter 20

Grief Savvy

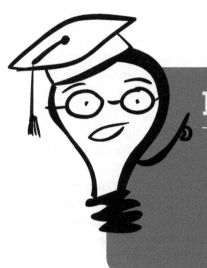

In This Chapter...

- What do we need to know about grief, mourning, and bereavement?
- What are the tasks of mourning?
- What is touch-and-go grief and mourning?
- What do we risk by not mourning our losses?

Grief is the normal response to a significant loss. However, grief feels anything *but* normal. Grieving is one of the hardest things we'll ever do in this life. Hence, we are wise to understand the process of grief and mourning so that we have realistic expectations of ourselves and others. Our society is fundamentally grief illiterate. Our lack of knowledge only serves to complicate the process and enhance our sense of loss. Being grief savvy will serve you and your family well when encountering the unavoidable losses of life.

In **Chapter 19**, we recognized that loss is a part of life. So we've all experienced the grief of loss numerous times. Why then are we apparently confused and confounded by grief? Essentially, we're afraid to discuss the subject of grief and loss. Because grief is typically associated with death, our fear of death and dying deters our exploration of the concept and process of grief. Consequently, we need to demystify the process by beginning with the basics—terminology. Once we know the language of grief, we can then discuss the process.

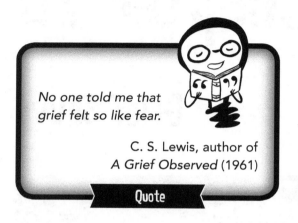

> No one told me that grief felt so like fear.
>
> C. S. Lewis, author of
> *A Grief Observed* (1961)
>
> **Quote**

Many of us grieve mightily, but we mourn poorly. This failure to mourn results in an accumulation of grief that weighs us down and holds us back. Unmourned loss is disabling. Consider our image of the bridge. Change happens. Something ends. We experience loss. Now we're standing at the entry point of the bridge, consumed by grief. The bridge provides the needed transition between what was and what will be. However, in order to move from one side to the other, we need to lighten our load. We need to get rid of our grief! The only way to do that is through the hard work of mourning. Feeling loss—*grief*—is one thing. Integrating loss—*mourning*—is something quite different. Understanding the distinction between grief and mourning is the first step in moving through and living beyond the significant losses of life. Mourning our losses moves us across the bridge toward a new way of being.

Basic Definitions

In order to discuss grief, mourning, and bereavement, we need to establish a common understanding of the terms. Quite often, the terms are used interchangeably. However, for the purpose of our discussion, the distinction between terms is necessary. This is not an easy task since the foundational terms are not universally understood or consistently defined by the recognized experts in the field of grief and bereavement. Granted, the variations are often subtle, but different nonetheless. Often the discrepancies and variations reflect the evolving nature of this field of study, *thanatology*.

Consequently, I offer basic definitions reflective of contemporary grief and bereavement experts. I will put a personal spin on the definitions predicated on my personal and professional experiences as well. You should know by now that I am all about applied learning. If it doesn't work in the trenches, it's of little use to me! So my definitions are a mix of theory and practice. With the definitional work completed, we'll then explore the hard work of grief and mourning.

Grief

Grief is our normal response to a significant loss. Most people think of a death loss when contemplating grief. But as noted in the previous chapter, we lose a variety of things over the course of a lifetime. If the loss is significant, we'll grieve. Grieving is the internal response to loss. It's the knot in our stomach. The lump in our throat. It's the tears that flow as sadness bubbles to the surface. Grief is how we *feel* about the loss. How we feel about the loss is then translated into thoughts and behaviors that inform how we experience and understand the loss.

You may have heard the terms normal grief and complicated grief. Normal grief is a process of anticipated phases/stages, emotions, and behaviors. Complicated grief is similar to normal grief with one important exception. With complicated grief, the intensity of emotions and duration of phases/stages are exacerbated.

If you remember nothing else from this chapter, remember this. We all grieve uniquely. There is no magical formula, template, path, or process that must be adhered to as you work through grief. However, understanding the general landscape of grief better prepares you for the arduous journey.

Mourning

If grief is how we *feel* about loss, mourning is what we *do* with loss. Mourning is the process of *doing* something with our emotions—internally and externally. It's the process of adapting to a world without the person or the thing we lost. We aren't just feeling the pain; we are

> ## Grief, Mourning, and Bereaved
>
> Grief is how we *feel* about loss. Mourning is what we *do* about loss. Bereaved is who we are and how we are after the death of a loved one.
>
> **Definition**

doing something about it. Funerals and memorial services often serve as the first step in the mourning process related to a death loss. It is the public declaration that we are grieving mightily because of a significant loss. This declaration is the invitation to other family members and friends to participate in and to support the mourning process. Mourning is a process of integration and adaptation. A challenging process indeed.

In the United States, we typically do a poor job of mourning. Our aversion to and ignorance of mourning are even reflected in corporate policies. How many days of bereavement leave does your employer allow? Usually only three days. Seriously? Do you honestly think it's realistic to expect a person to experience the death of a family member, attend the funeral, deal with the estate, express emotions, adapt to the loss, and return to work within three days? Hardly. However, due to corporate policies and societal norms, that's the expectation. Expectations inform our experience of grief, our own expectations, and the expectations of others. Hence, by understanding the experience of grief and mourning, we're able to establish more realistic expectations that actually encourage and support the process of mourning.

We also fail to mourn our losses due to fear and ignorance. We're afraid of the intensity of our emotions; we fear being consumed by our sadness and sorrow. So we opt to run away from our pain and avoid the hard work of adapting to the loss. We stuff our emotions—our grief—and hope the pain will fade away over time. Well, at some point, we learn that we can run but we can't hide. There will come a time when the flood gates of grief open and the sorrow of past losses washes over us. Instead of delaying the inevitable process of mourning, we are better served to confront the source of our pain and courageously mourn our losses. A bit later in the chapter, we'll chat about the personal costs of delayed mourning. We pay a high price, indeed, if we fail to mourn our losses.

Bereavement

Bereavement is a term typically associated with a death loss. It is a state of being caused by the death of a loved one. It should come as no surprise when I say that "loved one" includes people and critters in my world! Hospices and grief centers offer bereavement support groups for people who have experienced a death loss. At the end of the chapter, I'll discuss in greater detail available community resources for bereaved persons.

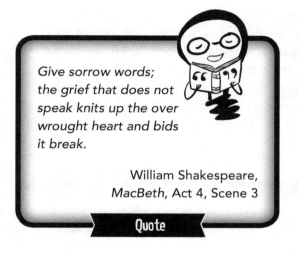

*Give sorrow words;
the grief that does not
speak knits up the over
wrought heart and bids
it break.*

William Shakespeare,
MacBeth, Act 4, Scene 3

Quote

Anticipatory Grief

Anticipatory grief is a type of grief all too familiar to caregivers and care receivers. E. Lindemann first described anticipatory grief in 1944 when studying the responses/reactions of couples dealing with terminal illness. He noted that the healthy spouse often began grieving the loss of their loved one well before the physical death. Anticipatory grief is the psychological and emotional reactions to an anticipated loss. Because grieving is hard work regardless of when we grieve, this is another aspect of caregiving that serves to exhaust the caregiver(s) and care receiver. Additionally, just because we grieve in anticipation of a loss doesn't mean our grief after the loss will be any easier. We must still do the hard work of integration and adaption after the loss.

Disenfranchised Grief

Disenfranchised grief is a grief not recognized or honored by society. Often people equate grief with the death of a family member or friend. Hence, any loss outside this limited perception is often diminished or discounted. Disenfranchised grief is often experienced in association with the death of a pet, partner, ex-spouse, nonfamily member, abortion, miscarriage, or nondeath losses. In order to compassionately support people who are grieving, we need to take the time to understand what a particular loss *means* to that person. We need not pass judgment on another's grief, deeming it worthy or not. Rather, we are called to compassionately companion those grieving the losses of life.

The *Hard* Work of Grief and Mourning

Grief and mourning are hard work. No way around it. After a significant loss, we can be and usually are emotionally distraught, physically exhausted, spiritually shaken, and mentally disoriented. For long-term caregivers, the grief over the death of a loved one compounds the exhaustion of caregiving. In the midst of grieving, we often feel confused because nothing seems normal. As we discussed in **Chapter 3**, we *long* for normal. But the harsh reality is this. You can't go back. The only option after a significant loss is to create a new normal. Not only is our world transformed by loss, but we are transformed as well. To reenter the world after a devastating loss, we must relearn and reengage the world in a different way. Our understanding of life is forever changed.

Example

Mourning on the Stairs

After my godfather died, I moved in with my godmother. I didn't want Aunt Jane to be alone as she adjusted to life without the love of her life. So I tried to fill a small portion of the huge void in her life. And in return, Aunt Jane taught me what courageous mourning looked like, sounded like, and felt like.

I remember the first night I heard her crying on the stairs. I was in the dining room studying for an exam the following day. At first, I didn't recognize the sound. And then I realized Aunt Jane was trying to muffle the sound of her crying so as not to disturb me. I walked to the foot of the stairs and looked up to see her huddled on the stairs leading to her bedroom. When she saw me, she started crying uncontrollably. I walked up the stairs, sat down, and wrapped my arms around her. We sat there for hours crying, talking, laughing, and just being. I had never witnessed such raw grief, such courage, and such determination. I had never seen Aunt Jane this vulnerable. It was concerning, frightening, and humbling all at the same time.

Every night after that, we met on the stairs at the same time to cry, talk, laugh, and be. At the time, I didn't realize or appreciate the gift of our time on the stairs. But today, I do. Aunt Jane taught me what it takes to mourn. Furthermore, she taught me that the pain of grief doesn't negate the eternal joy of having loved well. Needless to say, I learned more on the stairs than in class that semester.

Myths about Grief

How we engage the journey of grief and mourning depends on our expectations of the experience. Consequently, if your expectations are predicated on misinformation or myths about grief, the journey will be quite different than anticipated. Hence, you risk being ill prepared, reactive instead of proactive, and disillusioned. To avoid making a hard journey even harder, let's take the time to demystify grief and mourning. There are numerous misleading myths about grief that we accept as gospel because we lack the knowledge and/or experience to dispute. As always, knowledge is power. So, what is the truth about the journey of grief and mourning? Let's reveal the reality by discounting the common myths about grief and mourning.

Myth—Grief Occurs in a Linear Fashion

In *On Death and Dying* (1969), Elisabeth Kubler-Ross shared the results of her conversations with terminally ill patients. From her discussions, she identified five stages of dying: denial, bargaining, anger, depression, and acceptance. Her groundbreaking work in death and dying was then applied to grief and bereavement counseling. Although Kubler-Ross never intended for the stages to be perceived as a linear progression, that is exactly what happened. The public perception and subsequent expectation of grief was to begin with denial and end with acceptance, five stages resulting in closure. As such, people measured the progression of their journey against the Kubler-Ross standard. Over the years, numerous people have sought confirmation from me that their journey of grief was almost over because they were depressed. One more stage to go! Finish line in sight, right? Sorry, no. I couldn't provide the needed confirmation. But I could provide the much-needed grief education.

As we grieve and mourn, we will no doubt experience times of denial, bargaining, anger, depression, and acceptance. However, there is no predetermined sequence. You may start at acceptance after a long caregiving journey only to find yourself angry and raging at the fates in six months. Your journey unfolds uniquely depending on the circumstances of the loss. Additionally, the journey of grief is not linear by any means. Instead, it is best described as a spiral, a journey that doubles back and revisits previously experienced emotions and behaviors. Grieving is an iterative process. Some have likened grief to that of peeling an onion. Layer by layer, we go deeper into our grief. With each layer, we encounter the same emotions, but we respond differently as we continue to do the hard work of mourning.

Reality: Grief is not a linear process. My best advice is to feel what you feel when you feel it. Don't worry about where you are in the process. Resist seeking a finish line in the not-too-distant future. Remember, you will revisit a myriad of emotions as you work to integrate loss into your life.

Myth—You Will "Get Over" Grief

One of the most misleading and hurtful myths about grief is that we "get over" it. It's not uncommon for people to have an arbitrary time frame for grief. Perhaps the death of a spouse warrants a year of grief. Loss of job, maybe six months. Death of a pet? Just get another one! See what I mean? Expectations that serve no purpose but to make us feel as if we aren't grieving correctly. Why is it taking so long to "get over" my mom's death? Why am I so distraught over the death of my dog? This myth complicates the grieving process because it offers false hope. The myth offers the hope of a finish line. Our grief will end—sometime, someday. Sounds good, but it's not true. Best to know the reality of the journey before becoming mired in the muck of grief.

How could we possibly expect to "get over" the loss of someone or something we loved, cherished, and revered? How would that be possible? Yes, as we do the hard work of mourning, our pain changes. We round off the sharp edges of our emotions. But our sense of loss persists. How could it be otherwise?

Reality: Grief is a lifelong journey. We never "get over" a significant loss. Instead, we learn how to weave loss into the fabric of our lives. The hard work of mourning eventually results in the healing needed to appreciate the contrast provided by the dark threads (the losses) in our tapestry. This is a hard-earned view of life, a perspective that often transforms the way in which we choose to live and to engage future losses.

Myth—Time Heals All Wounds

I have forgotten many things over the years related to my mom's death and funeral. However, I do recall, with surprising clarity, the condolences offered by those in attendance. Over and over again, friends advised that time heals all wounds. "Just give it time. Things will get better." On that day, I desperately wanted to believe that time would heal my wounds. However, twelve years after my mom's death, I realized time alone heals nothing. If we choose to ignore the pain of our losses and therefore refuse to mourn, the wounds inflicted by loss persist and fester.

Reality: Time alone heals nothing. Our memory may dim a bit; however, the intensity of our grief persists until we do the hard work of mourning. Time *and* the hard work of mourning produce the healing balm needed by a grieving soul.

The Realities of Grief

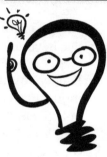

🔎 Grief is not a linear process. Don't worry about the stages of grief. Instead, feel what you feel when you feel it.

🔎 We never "get over" grief. Grief is a lifelong journey, a process of integrating loss into the fabric of our being.

🔎 Time alone heals nothing. Time and the hard work of mourning reduces the intensity of our pain.

🔎 Grief is counterintuitive. In order to heal, we must walk toward the source of our pain. There is no way around grief. We must move *through* our sorrow in order to live beyond it.

🔎 Grief is certainly personal, but it is rarely private. Loss affects the entire system in which we live. By allowing others to companion us in our grief, we share in the healing benefits of mourning.

🔎 Grief is not about "letting go." Rather, grief and the process of mourning are about the transformation of connections. Although a loved one may be physically absent, we still have the ability to connect through our memories, stories, and essence.

Myth—Run Away From the Source of Pain

Like most people, I'm not fond of pain. So, if something or someone is hurting me, I get as far away as possible! It's somewhat instinctual. Self-preservation. Perhaps that is why so many people run away from grief. Grief is painful, so we flee! We don't want to sit with our pain or confront the loss. Instead, we figure out a way to circumvent the grief. Or, if the pain is too great, we turn around and run in the opposite direction. Our hope is that by ignoring or delaying the process, our grief will diminish or fade away. However, grief doesn't have an expiration date.

Grief is counterintuitive. In order to grieve and mourn our losses, we must walk toward the source of our pain. The healing of mourning is possible only if we move *through* the pain. However, our natural inclination is to run away. It takes tremendous courage and conviction to confront the source of pain. Once confronted, we slowly resume control as we move through the pain to live beyond our loss.

Reality: Running away from grief only delays the needed process of mourning. Grief has an eternal shelf life. Hence, delaying the process serves only to clutter the corners of your heart. Discover the courage to confront your loss. Touch the wounds. Walk through the pain. And live beyond your sorrow. One step at a time.

Myth—Grief Is a Solitary Journey

We all grieve uniquely predicated on a variety of factors, which we'll discuss in the following section, Mediators of Mourning. Hence, grief is certainly a personal experience. However, grief is rarely private. We've noted numerous times that human beings are relational creatures. We enjoy the benefits and blessings of interdependent relationships. We affect and are affected by the systems in which we live. That means one person's loss affects the entire system to a greater or lesser extent. So, quite honestly, I feel your pain!

Although you may be at the epicenter of loss, there are others affected by the loss as well. Loss generates waves and ripples of grief that radiate throughout the system. Consequently, grief is not a solitary journey. You need not walk this path alone.

What Should I Say?

At times of tremendous loss, we often feel inept and inadequate. We don't know what to say to someone whose loved one died. What do you say to someone who just lost a job of twenty-five years? How do you console someone whose home was destroyed by a tornado? Perhaps if we realize there is *nothing* we can say to assuage the pain of loss, we'll feel less pressured to say anything. There is no *right* thing to say! At times of devastating loss, our courageous presence speaks volumes. Resist the temptation to offer lame platitudes that serve only to clutter the airwaves. Silence is golden. Just be present.

IMPORTANT!

Reality: Grief is personal, but rarely private. Often the journey is less daunting when companioned by those who understand our sense of loss and pain.

Myth—Grief Is About Letting Go

It was once thought that the task of the bereaved was to sever ties with the deceased in order to move on with life. Thank goodness that approach to grief counseling has evolved over the past fifty years! Grieving is not about severing relationships. Rather, it's about the transformation of relationships. Although our loved ones aren't physically present, we feel connected in different ways. We connect through memories. We connect by telling stories. We connect spiritually. My mom died thirty-two years ago. And yet I feel her presence every day. Yes, I would much prefer her physical presence. But that's not possible. So I am thankful beyond words for our eternal spiritual connection.

Reality: Grief is not about letting go. Grief is about learning how to reconnect in meaningful, life-giving ways.

Mediators of Mourning

With a significant loss, every member of your family will grieve and mourn uniquely. You may witness a wide variety of behaviors and emotional responses within your family related to the same loss. Why is that? Each person has a unique relationship with the person or the thing that was lost. The foundational work of Dr. J. William Worden, a respected authority in the field of grief and bereavement, highlights the determinants of our grief

No One Right Way to Mourn

When families experience a significant loss, tensions often arise due to differences in how family members grieve and mourn. There is no one right way to grieve and mourn. Allow each person to engage the journey of grief in his or her own, unique way. Honor, support, and respect each other. Resist directing the journey.

IMPORTANT!

response—the mediators of mourning. These are the factors that affect how loss is understood, experienced, and processed by individuals. Consider the following variables that determine the intensity, duration, and process of grief. For the purposes of this example, we'll assume grief is associated with a death loss. However, similar variables influence our response to any type of loss. You need only rephrase the questions to reflect the specific type of loss:

- *What was the relationship to the deceased?* Was the deceased a parent, child, sibling, friend, partner, or colleague? Was the relationship loving, contentious, abusive, conflicted, or estranged? How will the death of this person materially impact the bereaved?

- *What was the cause of death?* Was the death anticipated or unexpected? Did the deceased die of natural causes? Was the death violent? Is the cause of death stigmatized (such as suicide)? Is the death ambiguous (uncertainty as to whether the person is dead or alive)?

- *What is the bereaved's experience of loss?* Has the bereaved previously experienced a significant death loss? If so, was the previous loss adequately mourned? Or is the bereaved now faced with mourning multiple losses? What is the family legacy of grief and mourning?

- *What are the personal variables of the bereaved?* What are the age, gender, and ethnicity of the bereaved? How does the bereaved typically cope with loss? How or will the bereaved's foundational beliefs inform the journey of grief?

- *What support is readily available to the bereaved?* What social, family, and spiritual support is available to the bereaved?

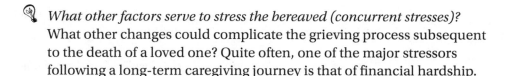 *What other factors serve to stress the bereaved (concurrent stresses)?* What other changes could complicate the grieving process subsequent to the death of a loved one? Quite often, one of the major stressors following a long-term caregiving journey is that of financial hardship.

Tasks of Mourning

In contrast to the stages of grief presented by Kubler-Ross in the 1960s, the tasks of mourning offer a more proactive approach for those who grieve. Describing each step as a *task* recognizes that mourning requires work. We must *do* something! In *Grief Counseling and Grief Therapy* (2008), Worden describes four tasks of mourning (a model developed in the 1990s). There are variations on the stages and/or tasks of mourning offered by other authorities in the field of grief and bereavement. However, Worden's work influenced most, if not all, of the subsequent models:

Accept the reality of loss. Now this sounds logical, right? However, grief is not always logical. Accepting the reality that a loved one died doesn't happen in a moment. Rather, it's a process of acceptance. The same is true for other significant losses as well. It takes time to cognitively accept the reality of loss.

Confront painful emotions. This particular task echoes our previous discussion about the realities of grief. In order to move through and beyond our sorrow, we must confront the pain of our loss. This requires incredible courage, conviction, and commitment.

Adapt to a changed world. In **Chapter 3**, we discussed at length the process of change and transition. We recognized that once a significant change/loss occurs, there is no going back. So we have a choice to make. We can choose to stand at the entry point of the bridge, paralyzed by fear and consumed by grief. Or we can choose to confront the pain of our loss, courageously mourn, adapt to our changed reality, and move across the bridge to embrace a new way of being. Crossing the bridge is a daunting proposition. We don't just skip across grinning from ear to ear! This is gut-wrenching, soul-stretching, belief-shaking, heartbreaking work. But if we are to survive the losses of life and ultimately thrive, we must do the hard work of mourning.

One step at a time, we cross the transitional bridge. Life will never be the same. And neither shall we.

 Transform the connection with the deceased and reengage life. When a loved one dies, we obviously lose the physical connection. However, our relationships entail more than physical contact. We remain connected through memories, stories, and spiritual presence. There

Shoes Are Gone

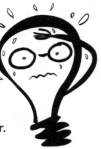

Shirley's husband of sixty years died six months ago. Not one to wallow in her emotions, Shirley decided to *do* something to move through the pain of his death. She cleaned out his closet and boxed up clothes for donation to her church and various agencies in town. Her husband had always been a snappy dresser. How he loved his suits and silk ties! Now someone else would be looking dapper in those same suits.

Although the process of sorting his clothes brought back countless memories, Shirley said she did well until she got to her husband's shoes. His Italian, leather loafers were his pride and joy. As she stood there considering the various options, she said out loud, "I can't give his shoes away. When he comes home, he'll kill me!" As she related this story to me, she asked for confirmation that she had officially crossed the line. She *had* lost her mind! After six months, she *knew* her husband wasn't coming back home. And yet she spoke those words. When I refused to confirm her believed state of insanity, she then asked for a directive. She wanted to be *told* to give the shoes away. Again, I refused to comply. Instead, I advised her to be gentle with herself in the process of grief and mourning. She didn't have to do it all in one day. As for the shoes, she would give them away when she was ready.

I saw Shirley four months later. A woman of few words, she updated me in short order. "Shoes are gone." And so was Shirley shortly thereafter. The grief support group had served her well. She was now ready to get on with the task of living. We all accept the reality of loss in our own time and in our own way. One step at a time.

are countless reminders of our loved ones if we have eyes to see and ears to hear. Immediately following the death of a loved one, the reminders are often quite painful. However, with time and the hard work of mourning, the reminders serve to reinforce our spiritual connections with those who have died. Then the challenge becomes reengaging life and reinvesting ourselves in other people.

Touch-and-Go Grief and Mourning

The Ordinary Things Are the Hardest

It's the ordinary things that are the hardest after the death of a loved one. The ordinary, yet sacred, routines that we too often take for granted. How do you start the day without sharing a cup of coffee and the paper with your beloved? What will it feel like to be single again after being a couple for fifty years? What will it be like to walk through my neighborhood without my beloved dog, Bella, walking by my side? Well, it will be different. And it will be hard. And it will be sad. It's the ordinary things that are the hardest after the death of a loved one. So, today, cherish the ordinary blessings in your life. These are sacred times indeed.

Example

Mourning is a complex process of adaptation that is often unpredictable. We all grieve and mourn uniquely, in our own way and in our own time. However, there is one thing I know to be true about grief and mourning. It is a *touch-and-go* process, very similar to learning how to land an airplane.

Several years ago, I watched student pilots practicing "touch-and-go" landings. The plane would touch down on the runway for a short time. Then the plane would take off again. Touch and go. The pattern was repeated over and over again. Witnessing this process, I realized how similar learning to land a plane is to grieving.

As noted previously, grief is a lifelong journey. We never get over our grief. We never fully mourn our losses. Instead, we touch and go. I may awaken tomorrow and *land* on the pain of my mom's death. I will *touch* that grief for a period of time, and then I'll *go*. Each time I land on the pain of my loss, I'll touch that grief in a little bit different way. From a little bit different perspective. Because each time I

Lilacs in the Spring

Every spring, my mom and I conducted a lovely lilac ritual. When our lilac bush bloomed, we poured a glass of iced tea and grabbed a lawn chair. We then sat beside the lilac bush and enjoyed the familiar fragrance as we talked about life. Growing up in Ohio, my mom enjoyed fields of lilacs in the spring. So the fragrance brought back many a childhood memory that she shared with me.

The first spring following my mom's death, the familiar fragrance of lilacs ignited an overwhelming surge of grief. It literally brought me to my knees, tears streaming down my face. The pain was almost more than I could bear, or so I thought.

Now, thirty-two years later, the fragrance of lilacs still brings tears to my eyes every spring. But, they are tears of joy instead of sorrow. I am reminded of the constant presence of my mom. I rejoice in the amazing bond we shared and continue to share. I remember the times we welcomed and celebrated the coming of spring. The fabulous fragrance of lilacs once again signals the promise of renewal, growth, and life. A lovely, timeless connection to my mom.

Pure Genius!

touch my grief, I bring something different to the experience. As I change and evolve as a person, I perceive and experience my grief differently. Integration of loss into our lives is a touch-and-go process. Such is the nature of mourning.

The Need to Mourn Our Losses

We've established that grief is a normal response to a significant loss in life. Grief is how we *feel* about loss. Mourning, on the other hand, is what we *do* about loss. Mourning is the process of courageously confronting our pain, walking across the transitional bridge, and choosing to reengage life. If we fail to mourn our losses, grief persists and accumulates over time. Our grief serves to restrict our ability and willingness to incur the risks of future loss. We don't want to feel any more pain. We can't handle any more grief. So we isolate. Isolation certainly reduces the risk of loss. However, in like fashion, isolation limits the possibility of fulfillment.

Far too often, we grieve mightily and mourn poorly. Some signs of unmourned losses include the following:

- Fear of change
- Heightened anxiety
- Loss of purpose
- Emotional numbness
- Disengagement
- Lack of joy
- Fear of intimacy
- Depression

If we fail to recognize the signs of unmourned loss and subsequently fail to address our burden of grief, we risk the overwhelming task of mourning multiple losses at some future time. We can carry only so much grief before the pressure becomes unbearable. Why wait for the dam to break? We needn't experience a catastrophic flood of painful emotions. Instead, we can manage the flow of grief by intentionally mourning our losses, one at a time. Remember, proactive trumps reactive *every* time!

Grief Resources

When grieving, many people benefit from community and online grief resources. Medicare requires that all hospice organizations provide bereavement services for patients and families. Additionally, many hospices provide bereavement services to the greater community as well. Individual grief counseling as well as grief support groups may be available in your community through a local hospice. Check with your local hospice providers to determine the availability and associated costs of bereavement services. Outside of hospice, grief support is provided by funeral homes, grief centers, faith communities, and individual grief counselors.

The Internet is a rich resource for grief education as well as grief support. The Association of Death Education and Counseling (adec.org) is a membership organization that provides a variety of educational resources to members. The Hospice Foundation of America (hospicefoundation.org) is another fabulous resource for grief education. Both organizations provide foundational and current information about grief and bereavement. Online grief support is quite popular due to its convenience and

Remember How to Mourn

- See the loss— recognize the loss.

- Speak the loss—articulate feelings, emote.

- Sit with the loss—confront the pain.

- Share the loss—reach out to others.

- Spiritualize the loss—ritualize the loss.

- Synthesize the loss—integrate loss into life.

Pure Genius!

24/7 availability. One note of caution. If confidentiality is of concern to you, be sure to confirm exactly how the groups are conducted, managed, and monitored. Not all grief support groups are created equal. Based on your particular loss, you will no doubt be able to find an online support group.

To Summarize...

- Grief is the normal response to a significant loss. Grief is how we *feel* about the loss. Mourning is what we *do* about the loss. And bereaved is who we are and how we are after the death of a loved one.

- We typically grieve mightily and mourn poorly. Unmourned losses serve to weigh us down and hold us back. We often resist mourning our losses out of fear or ignorance. Hence, knowledge is power. We need to understand the process of mourning in order to integrate loss into our lives.

- There are many myths about grief that have been handed down from generation to generation. Our experience of grief is often predicated on our expectations of grief. Many of the myths serve to derail and complicate the process of grief and mourning. Knowing the reality of grief gets us back on track.

- There is no one right way to grieve. We will all grieve and mourn uniquely predicated on the mediators of mourning.

- Grief is one of the hardest experiences of life. Keep in mind, we need not grieve and mourn in isolation. There are numerous community and online resources available to assist those challenged by loss. Grief education and grief support can be incredibly beneficial for all types of loss. Seek the information and the help you need and desire. Become grief savvy. It will serve you and yours well.

Chapter 21

The Reality of Mortality

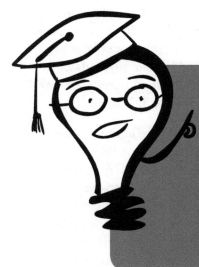

In This Chapter...

- How does awareness of our mortality enhance the lived experience?
- What informs our attitudes about death and dying?
- What can we expect at the end of the road?
- Why should we *bother* with end-of-life rituals?

Quite often, the terminating event of the caregiving journey is the death of the care receiver. The ultimate loss. Since we live in a death-averse society, the specter of death overshadows the journey to the end of the road. We are scared to death of death! Our reluctance to confront the reality of our mortality inhibits our ability to be fully present to the moment. Since this is a once-in-a-lifetime opportunity, how can we better prepare ourselves for the end of the road?

Our experience of death certainly informs our attitudes about death and dying. Our cultural, societal, family, and spiritual norms also contribute to our understanding of death. Did your family speak openly about death and dying when you were a child? Did you attend funerals and memorial services? Have you been present at the bedside when someone died?

For many people, death happens at a distance. In the hospital. At a care center. On the big screen. Through the media. Death is not intimate. So we don't know what death looks like, sounds like, smells like, and feels like. And what we don't know frightens us. Thus, once again, knowledge is power. By understanding what to expect physically, emotionally, spiritually, and psychosocially, we are no longer disabled by fear. Instead, we are free to engage *life* and courageously walk to the end of the road.

> At some point in life—sometimes in youth, sometimes late—each of us is due to awaken to our mortality.
>
> Irvin D. Yalom, MD, author of *Staring at the Sun: Overcoming the Terror of Death* (2008), Emeritus Professor of Psychiatry at Stanford University
>
> **Quote**

Death, as the ultimate loss, is a major destabilizing event in the life of a family. Upon the death of a loved one, we long for normalcy and some sense of control. We need an anchor in our storm of grief and mourning, something known and trusted that keeps us from drifting out to sea. Ritual often serves as that important anchor. Historically, we have relied on end-of-life rituals to restore a sense of continuity, connection, and meaning. Never doubt the importance and significance of end-of-life rituals. However you choose to ritualize the ultimate loss, it *is* worth the bother.

Life as a Terminal Condition

Have you ever thought about life as a terminal condition? I think this is worthy of consideration for a variety of reasons. First, because it's true! We are all born with an expiration date; we just don't know exactly when our time's up. But we do know that our time is limited. Or we *should* know. Second, if we perceive life as time delimited, we're more apt to appreciate the moment. There is no guarantee as to how many more moments we get. So enjoy this one! When there is a limited supply, the commodity becomes much more precious. Supply and demand. Pretty simple.

What if I told you today was the last day of your life? What would you do on your final day in this world? How would you spend your final twenty-four hours? With whom would you share your final moments? Interesting proposition, eh? Kind of fun to discuss with family and friends. Exploring the what-ifs. But what if today really *was* the last day of your life? Are you currently living as if you had all the time in the world, or are you living as if your time is limited? Are you just going through the motions, or are you fully engaged in life?

This is why death is so important to the journey of life. Knowing that we will die informs how we intentionally choose to live. Accepting, instead of rejecting, the fact that we'll die enhances the sacredness of each moment lived. We become more appreciative of life. And that is a very good thing indeed! Our mortality gives meaning and purpose to our existence. Knowing the journey could end at any moment motivates us to be present to the *now*. To be present to each other. To squeeze the *life* out of life! Knowing our time is limited adds a sense of urgency to the journey. The reality is that we will all die; we are mortal. However, we need not fear death. Rather, we should fear never having lived fully.

My work as a hospice chaplain and educator transformed my perceptions of life and death. Ironic, isn't it, that by companioning people who were dying, I learned how to live? I learned how I wanted to live. Intentionally. Courageously. Present. Engaged. Grateful. I also learned that our fear of death serves only to sap our energy, divert our attention, and inhibit our ability to live in the moment. The fact of the matter is that we'll all die. That is one of the givens in life. The real challenge is to *live* until we die. Far too many people die before they are dead! Don't allow the fear of death to derail your journey. There is much to be seen, to be done, to be heard, to be felt, and to be spoken as we take those final steps. Embrace the moments. Live until you die.

The subject of death is daunting for most people. For the majority of my life, I was paralyzed by the prospect of death. And because of that, I missed once-in-a-lifetime opportunities at the end of the road with family members and friends. With the help of some amazing friends and mentors, I eventually confronted my fears about death and dying. Today, I'm not fearless. But I'm no longer fearful. I have a different understanding and appreciation of

Fly and Be Free!

Many years ago, I spent a day traversing a high-ropes course and emerged transformed. It was an obstacle course constructed thirty-five feet off the ground in a wooded area of eastern Oklahoma. Quite the adventure since I have a fear of heights! However, it was exactly the challenge I needed and wanted. As the day unfolded, I climbed higher and reached farther than I ever imagined. I completed the entire course with the encouragement of my friends and instructor. Confronting our fears usually requires some coaching and sustaining support.

As we were basking in the glow of our accomplishments, the instructors offered one final challenge. The Pamper Pole, a thirty-five-foot vertical telephone pole. We were to climb the pole. Somehow stand on top. Then leap from the pole to a trapeze bar seven feet out from the pole. Simple enough, right? Well, simple if you aren't afraid of heights!

As I watched several people scale the pole and successfully complete the challenge, I doubted my ability to replicate their success. But I knew I would regret not trying. So, before logic prevailed, I started up the pole. The hardest part was standing on top of the pole. Letting go and rising up. But once done, I saw life in a totally different way. I felt like a totally different person. My fear of heights had not prevented me from engaging and enjoying this day. I had overcome my fear. And I felt incredibly free! As I eyed the trapeze bar swinging seven feet in front of me, I knew I wouldn't miss. This was my time to fly and be free. So I soared!

That day on the Pamper Pole taught me an invaluable life lesson. We can choose to live in fear or in spite of fear. By overcoming our fear, we are free to jump at the opportunities presented by life. Don't get me wrong. I still have a healthy respect for heights. But my fear no longer holds me back. Once you've experienced life from atop the Pamper Pole, you won't easily relinquish that perch. The view is spectacular!

mortality. Death is not a threat; it's the reality of humanity. We will all die. Knowing that, the question then becomes how we choose to live. Today, I *see* life differently. I have a different perspective derived from experience, knowledge, and age. Death now enhances my appreciation of the moment. Knowing what I have to lose compels me to *jump* at the chance to live!

By accepting the reality that death is part of life, we are able to experience all that the end of the road has to offer. Please, please, please don't miss this opportunity. Be prepared for the end of the road. A good place to start in the preparatory process is identifying your attitudes and perceptions of death and dying. Attitudes that serve you well, retain. Those that don't, reject or transform.

Attitudes about Death and Dying

Our attitudes about death and dying are informed and influenced by societal, cultural, family, and spiritual norms. Additionally, our experiences of death—or lack thereof—serve to shape our perceptions of death as well. The combination of factors determines whether we are more or less anxious about death. For many, the greater concern is the manner of death, not death itself. In order to mitigate any fears we have about death and dying, we must identify the source of our angst. So let's review the major influences.

Societal Attitudes and Norms

Death has historically been an enigma. Try as we might, human beings are incapable of understanding everything there is to know about death. Consequently, it's the "unknown" that gets the juices flowing, the heart fluttering, and the imagination bubbling. Human beings have always been and will always be perplexed by death. However, we love a good mystery, don't we? Beginning with the oldest known book about death, *The Egyptian Book of the Dead*, dated at 1240 BC, we've attempted to demystify death and guide people through the dying process. And yet, despite the valiant efforts of many, death remains a mystery. When the body ceases to function, what then?

Philippe Ariès published a book in 1982, *The Hour of Our Death*, in which he reviewed the evolution of death attitudes in Western society. It's a fascinating overview of the historical dance between spiritual beliefs, societal evolution, global events, medical advances, and death attitudes. Over the past three thousand years, we've evolved in amazing and miraculous ways. Consider the technology and the medical advances available today that weren't even imagined a century ago. And yet we still struggle to define when life begins and when life ends. The mystery remains.

Today, death is perceived as unacceptable. With all of the available medical interventions, we can keep death at bay. Right? Well, as we all know, not indefinitely. But that doesn't keep us from trying. Just consider the time, talents, and treasures expended on a daily basis in an attempt to avoid death. We are so busy fighting off death that we fail to live. It's the old story of rearranging the deck chairs on the Titanic as the ship went down. Instead of confronting the reality of the situation—death—we distract ourselves with less daunting tasks. Consequently, we miss the moment. Admittedly, it takes tremendous courage to go down with the ship—to walk to the end of the road. But this is the reality of life. We are much better served to accept the reality of our mortality than to continue the futile struggle of denying death. Choose your battles wisely. Always good advice.

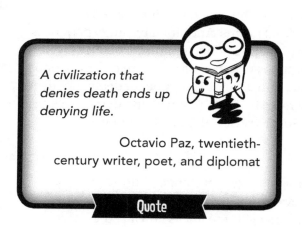

A civilization that denies death ends up denying life.

Octavio Paz, twentieth-century writer, poet, and diplomat

Quote

Family Norms and Cultural Norms

Family and cultural norms heavily influence individual attitudes regarding death and dying. Think of your own family. Are your attitudes about death and dying reflective of the attitudes of your parents and grandparents? Are your attitudes similar to those of people within your faith community, neighborhood, or social setting? More than likely, your attitudes reflect the influence of your family and cultural influences to a great extent.

With that said, we need to consider if our family norms serve us well. As we noted in **Chapter 5** in our discussion about the family legacy of caregiving, we can choose to perpetuate or to transform our family legacies. For example, in my family, we did not speak about death. Even though my mom was diagnosed with a terminal illness, we never spoke of the possibility of death during the eight years of surgeries and treatments. At least I wasn't aware of any discussions. Perhaps my parents chose to protect me from the harsh reality of death, opting to discuss death privately. Regardless, I was not privy to a discussion about death and, therefore, was not prepared for my mom's death. Consequently, my initial experience of a significant death was traumatizing. The reticence of my family to talk about death did not serve me well. As evidenced by my current passion for end-of-life care, I have transformed my family legacy related to death and dying. I do speak about death. And the transformation serves me well.

In addition to family norms, cultural norms inform our attitudes about death and dying. Remember from **Chapter 5**, culture is everything that makes you *you*! So consider the myriad of factors that affect your perceptions of death. Do these cultural norms related to death serve you well? Cultural sensitivity and respect is necessary when discussing death and dying. Within some cultures, it is inappropriate and disrespectful to speak of death. In fact, to speak of death is to invite death. There are other cultures in which the subject of death may be broached with family members but not with the person who is dying. As you might imagine, there are differences between cultures and within cultures as to how death is perceived, discussed, and understood. Although fascinating, my intent is not to exhaustively discuss the cultural variations. Rather, I want to encourage the examination of our cultural roots related to our perception of death. Feed the cultural roots that provide life-giving nutrients. Trim the ones that don't.

Your Experience of Death

Do you remember your first experience of death? Most people do. We remember because the experience of death changes our understanding of life. Perhaps we no longer feel safe. Life seems uncertain or frightening. We feel exposed, vulnerable, and at risk. The circumstances surrounding the death are incredibly important as well. How old were you? Who or what died? Was the death tragic or violent? Did anyone talk to you about the death? Did you attend a funeral or memorial service? All the details related to the first death serve to define your initial experience of death. Good or bad, that initial experience becomes a lifelong memory that either helps or hinders you with future losses.

Today, because people are living longer, many people don't experience a significant death loss until they're adults. I was relatively young when my parents died. Twenty-four when my mom died. Forty-one when my dad died. Although my friends were incredibly supportive at the time, none had experienced a similar loss. Consequently, they had a different perspective of death than I. Whether child or adult, our experience of death reshapes our view of life *and* death. We are forever changed.

I want to highlight something of importance related to children and death. Children understand death based on their level of cognitive development. Until a child can think concretely and understand abstract concepts (around the age of seven), the finality of death is elusive. So children will experience and grieve death quite differently from adults. If you are desirous of more information about children, grief, and loss, I highly recommend The Dougy Center (dougy.org). This organization offers resources, information, and counseling for grieving children and families.

Faith

In **Chapter 9**, we discussed spirituality and religion. At that point, I opted to avoid the major debate of terminology and declared I would use "faith" as the all-encompassing term for foundational beliefs. As such, faith certainly informs our understanding of death and attitudes toward death. If you believe that life is in preparation for a better existence yet to come, the prospect of death may not be frightening. In fact, you may view death as

It Could Happen to Me

When I was in second grade, I remember going to school one day and noticing the absence of a classmate, Mark. The remarkable thing about his absence was that his desk had been emptied and his name removed from his locker. After three days, I thought to mention this to my mom. I remember the sadness in her eyes. She told me that Mark had been killed in a car accident while on vacation with his parents over the holidays. I was shocked! I asked how she knew this, and she showed me the obituary in the newspaper. I remember his picture in the paper so well. He looked so alive! And yet, he was dead. It dawned on me as I read his obituary that he was *my* age! If that could happen to Mark, it could happen to me. Suddenly, I felt very scared. I didn't feel as safe as I once did.

Example

your final reward. However, if you fear the repercussions of a sinful life, death is the herald of eternal punishment and suffering. If so, the prospect of death generates a great deal of anxiety and fear. Or perhaps you perceive death as the end. There is nothing beyond the end of the road. The only existence you need to be concerned about is this one. Consequently, there is no need to look beyond the end of the road. The focus is on the here and now. Just from these three examples, it's obvious that our beliefs (faith) inform our experience at the end of the road.

Faith not only informs our understanding and perception of death and dying; faith also serves to support and sustain us as we experience the ultimate loss of life. When we need a port in the storm, our faith is often the light that guides us to safe harbor. Our guiding principles and beliefs provide a sense

IMPORTANT!

It's a Mystery

When I walked into Anne's room, I could tell something was up. After working with her for nine months, I recognized when she had something of concern on her heart and mind. As I sat down, she took my hand and looked directly at me. She asked, "What do you think Heaven is like?" I knew Anne wanted reassurance as to what she would encounter at the end of the road. We had explored this concern many times over the past few months. And each time, I responded in the same way. "I don't know. It's a mystery." And each time, Anne would furrow her brow and groan in disgust! As her spiritual director, she expected an answer. Today was no different in that regard. However, I sensed she was ready to move beyond her disgust with me and explore her question a bit further. So I turned the tables on her. I asked, "What do *you* think Heaven is like?" And that's when Anne threw me a curveball. I think she had been saving it for months. She looked at me with a funny smile and said, "Beats me! You're the spiritual director. If you don't know, how should I?" And with that, we enjoyed a good laugh that was a mystery to everyone up and down the hall. Sometimes you just need a good belly laugh as you walk to the end of the road. Helps to keep things in perspective.

of purpose and control that we so desperately need as we walk to the end of the road. Our faith provides the solid foundation from which we courageously confront our fears of death and dying. We are all guided by a unique light and will consequently have a unique experience as we walk to the end of the road.

Death Awareness

Our society would be even more death averse were it not for the pioneers in end-of-life care noted previously in **Chapter 11**. Elisabeth Kubler-Ross and those involved in the development of hospice and palliative care services in the United States initiated the conversation about death and dying. We've realized that by shining the spotlight on death and discussing the reality of our mortality, the specter of death is less frightening. By naming and addressing our fear, we can disarm death. Yes, we will ultimately die. But we need not be scared to death in the process! We owe the pioneers in death and dying our *undying* gratitude. Because of their groundbreaking work, we are better prepared to walk to the end of the road with our eyes wide open. We can choose to live until we die.

The End of the Road

I have walked to the end of the road several times with family (people and critters), friends, and patients. I have walked the road as a companion. Not as the principal. Hence, I have only a limited perspective of the journey. With each journey, I have grown in my capacity to be present to the moment, to be present to life. This, I believe, is one of the most challenging aspects of companioning someone to the end of the road. It's hard to be fully present when we're an emotional wreck! We distract ourselves with the minutiae of care—straightening the sheets, preparing appetizing food, offering sips of water or ice chips, checking monitors, administering medications, and countless other things. I am not diminishing the need for some of these activities. But sometimes I think we do all these things to avoid the journey. To avoid looking at death. But, as we noted earlier, if we confront our fear of death, we disarm death. We need to find the courage to stare death down, for ourselves and for those we companion. In order to overcome our fears, we need to know what to expect as companions and as the principal. What will happen physically, emotionally, psychosocially, and spiritually as we approach the end of the road?

Physical Changes

At the end of the road, the body begins the natural process of slowing down all functions. Every person will move through the process at a different pace, but the process is fairly predictable. By knowing what to expect, the dying process is less frightening for those companioning the dying person. As a person approaches the end of the road, you can expect to witness the following physical changes:

- Sleepiness, semiconsciousness
- Difficulty swallowing
- Congestion in the lungs
- Loss of appetite
- Bladder and bowel incontinence
- Changes in breathing
- Cool extremities
- Smell—acetone odor
- Discoloration of the skin
- Possible agitation or restlessness
- Eventual unconsciousness

Spiritual Changes

Spiritual changes are much less predictable than the physical changes of the dying. There is really no way to know whether a person's sense of the sacred will be enhanced or diminished by the experience of death. I have seen both extremes and everything in between. So one size definitely does not fit all.

However, the one thing that is seemingly universal about the journey to the end of the road is the desire to "remember when." We have a tremendous need to reflect on the lived experience. And we need people who are willing and able to participate in the process. It's important for all of us to reflect on our lives and discern a sense of meaning and purpose. To recognize the footprints we left in the sand. We need to believe that our life mattered. That we made a difference in the world. This *is* a spiritual process since the function and purpose of our foundational beliefs is the search for significance. Our foundational beliefs help us answer the big whys of life. Well, there is no greater *why* than "Why was I here?" To be a part of this conversation is sacred indeed. There is much to be learned by listening well. And it is one of the greatest gifts we have to offer the dying, and they to us.

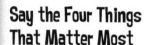

Say the Four Things That Matter Most

Please forgive me. I forgive you. Thank you. I love you.

Ira Byock, MD, Director of Palliative Medicine at Dartmouth–Hitchcock Medical Center (2003 through July 2013), author of *The Four Things that Matter Most* (2004)

Quote

Psychosocial Changes

We have noted the challenges of role changes many times in our discussion of caregiving. As we succumb to advanced age or a serious illness, we're no longer able to fulfill various roles within the family. Our relationships change. We see ourselves differently. We are seen differently. We assume the new role of care receiver and rely on others for basic aspects of care.

These psychosocial changes continue as the journey progresses. One change that often concerns families is that care receivers can become withdrawn and less social. There's a greater desire and need for solitude and quiet reflection. Quite often, family members interpret this introspective behavior as a sign of depression. However, for some people, it is the natural process of disengaging from this existence in preparation for death.

As we prepare for death, there is often the need or desire to heal old wounds or mend fences with family and friends. We want to exit this lifetime with a clear conscience if possible. Even if forgiveness is not possible, perhaps reconciliation is. I have witnessed some amazing reunions as well as devastating rejections. It just depends on the specifics of the estrangement and the willingness of both parties to reunite.

Many families struggle with crowd control at the end of life. Who needs to be there? Who wants to be there? Who shouldn't be there? Whether a person chooses to be surrounded by family and friends at the time of death is often reflective of how the person lived. However, there isn't always a one-to-one correlation. If the person is capable of articulating a preference, it is best to ask.

Emotional Changes

As we approach the end of the road, we often have a tremendous urge to say things we've never said before. This is true for caregivers *and* care receivers. We want to express our love, gratitude, pride, and appreciation to those who have meant the most to us. We want to make sure our loved ones know how we feel before it's too late. But we often hesitate because it's too hard. We don't want to upset our loved ones. Or we think we have more time. We'll say it tomorrow. Well, here's the mantra to remember as you walk to the end of the road. Say what you need to say—and say it *right now*. There is no guarantee you'll have tomorrow to share what's on your heart.

In **Chapter 20**, we explored the journey of grief and mourning, so I won't belabor the issue here. However, it's important to remind family members that the care receiver is grieving as well. In fact, the burden of grief is often greater for the dying person than for the survivors. Think about it. How many people, places, critters, and things must the dying bid adieu? The survivors must say goodbye to one person. The dying person is losing an entire family, community, home, career, and life! So, even though family members may not be able and willing to explore the grief of the care receiver, find someone who can and will. Perhaps a trusted friend who is not as distraught as the immediate family members. Maybe a pastoral care provider. Chaplain. Spiritual director. Grief counselor. If the care receiver expresses the need and desire to talk, find a capable and compassionate person who will listen well. This is a gift indeed.

Often what the dying need most is our presence. The dying need someone who is courageous enough to be present to whatever is in the room. Plain and simple. They need our courageous presence and our willingness to listen to and discuss their fears, their hopes, and their grief. The dying need to talk about dying! However, too often we're afraid to listen. We're afraid to have the poignant conversation. Having been afraid, I missed this sacred opportunity with both my mom and dad. I invite you to benefit from my experience.

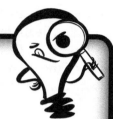

Death Avoided— Ivan Ilych

Leo Tolstoy tells the timeless story of death aversion in his book *The Death of Ivan Ilych* (1886). Ivan, diagnosed with a terminal illness, is most distressed by his family's unwillingness to talk about his imminent death. Instead, everyone acts as if Ivan will eventually recover. His greatest source of suffering is his inability to discuss the fact that he is dying. He is forced to take part in a lie that all will be well. When, in fact, he knows it will not. He knows he is dying. His only source of solace comes in the form of a peasant boy, Gerasim, who is quite comfortable speaking of death. Living on a farm, the young boy witnesses life and death on a daily basis. Death is not a stranger to the boy. Death is not something to be feared. Death is part of life. So Gerasim courageously and compassionately companions Ivan to the end of the road. Something Ivan's family is unable to do. A missed blessing for both Ivan and his family.

Definition

Don't miss walking to the end of the road with those you love. Have no regrets.

End-of-Life Rituals

In **Chapter 3**, we discussed the importance of ritual in the midst of change. If you'll recall, we said that ritual is a prescribed set of actions involving symbolic elements. The purpose of ritual is to provide a sense of continuity, connection, and meaning for those engaged in the process. Ritual provides a sense of certainty, normalcy, and predictability that we need and want when everything else is beyond our control. So, with that said, wouldn't ritual be a fabulous thing when we're confronted by the ultimate loss? Absolutely!

So let's explore how and why end-of-life rituals serve us so well. This includes funerals, memorials, and other rites deemed beneficial as we travel to the end of the road. Some rituals may be conducted prior to death. Some rituals are conducted after death. Regardless, end-of-life rituals serve to facilitate the process of change and transition. Rituals help with the integration of loss into life going forward. At the end of the road, we *hunger* for ritual.

Historical Importance of Ritual

There is historical evidence of death rituals dating back to 60,000 BC.

Archeological excavations of Neanderthal remains show evidence of some sort of ritual. Fossilized flowers. Pieces of shells. Items that indicate an honoring of the deceased. So end-of-life rituals are nothing new. Human beings have historically sought ways to honor the dead, tame our fears about death and dying, and regain a sense of normalcy and control. Rituals are timeless, as is our need for order, healing, integration, meaning, and community during times of loss.

Function of End-of-Life Ritual

There's been a great deal of debate recently regarding the relevance of funerals and memorial services. In fact, some critics have accused the Boomer generation and subsequent generations of turning our backs on ritual altogether. As we become a more secular culture, there appears to be less adherence to the traditional, religious rituals of past generations. However, I would argue that ritual is still of tremendous importance.

Today, ritual is often "done" differently and not recognized as such by some of the critics. However, not everyone resonates with a traditional funeral or memorial service. People are choosing to put a personal spin on ritual, thus making the experience more meaningful for those involved. Additionally, we now have technological options that have transformed ritual in a variety of ways. We'll discuss some contemporary forms of ritual in the following section about technology and rituals.

The one thing we need to understand is that ritual evolves and changes over time in concert with societal evolution and change. That is to be expected. If ritual is to fulfill the promise of providing connection, continuity, and meaning, the ritual must resonate with the person or community conducting the ritual. The ritual must be relevant. So the symbols, elements, and platform of ritual may change over time, but our need for ritual remains the same.

Today, as in prehistoric times, we need end-of-life rituals to facilitate the transition after a death loss. An end-of-life ritual serves in the following ways:

- Acts as the last rite of passage for the deceased

- Highlights the reality of mortality

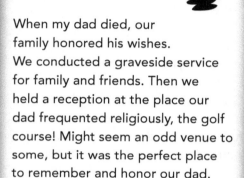

Par for the Course

When my dad died, our family honored his wishes. We conducted a graveside service for family and friends. Then we held a reception at the place our dad frequented religiously, the golf course! Might seem an odd venue to some, but it was the perfect place to remember and honor our dad.

As the reception was winding down, one of my friends suggested we go to the driving range and hit some balls in my dad's honor. What a fabulous tribute! I ran to my car and pulled out my dad's golf clubs. We all took a club and grabbed a bucket of balls as we headed to the driving range. In the fading light of that November evening, I'm sure my dad took great delight in the sendoff provided by family and friends. I'm also sure he was equally delighted to see my drives flying straight and true. He and I spent a lot of time trying to straighten out my slice. Better late than never!

Pure Genius!

- Initiates the mourning process
- Stimulates stories of the deceased
- Honors a life lived
- Allows the community to participate in mourning
- Comforts the bereaved
- Contributes to the process of integration of loss
- Facilitates understanding and the search for meaning
- Affirms the social order

Technology and Rituals

The manner in which we communicate and relate has changed dramatically over the past twenty years. Yes, this is me stating the obvious once again! But what may not be quite as obvious is how communication technology has transformed and continues to transform the way in which we conduct and experience end-of-life rituals. Think about the last funeral or memorial service you attended. Was the service videotaped? Live streamed? Posted on YouTube? Was there a digital photo album? Did you see a video clip of the deceased? Did people post pictures of the service on their Facebook page? Tweet from the reception? Send a text while in the service? I am sure you witnessed some if not all of these forms of communication.

We also use the Internet as a platform for ritual. There are online virtual memorial and cemetery websites. Websites for individuals or communities (communal losses such as 9/11) provide the opportunity for visitors to post messages, upload pictures and videos, and offer condolences. If you are interested in these sites and services, Google the following terms: online cemeteries, online obituaries, and online memorials. These are sites that invite people to participate in a type of virtual ritual honoring those who died. Yes, it's quite different from the traditional rituals of most faith traditions. However, it's ritual nonetheless.

One of the benefits of online memorials and cemeteries is that the opportunity to participate is unlimited. The sites are available 24/7 from anywhere in the world. Hence, if you are unable to attend the physical funeral, you can always participate virtually via an online site. Online ritual serves the same historical human need during times of loss. Rituals of all kinds help us heal.

Is Ritual Worth the *Bother?*

We initially started this conversation about caregiving by noting the changing nature of families. We noted how the changes in contemporary families (smaller, geographically dispersed, etc.) complicate the caregiving journey oftentimes. Well, those same changes can complicate the process of ritual at the end of life. When families are scattered across the globe, is it feasible to expect family members to attend the funeral? With the extraordinary health care costs associated with the caregiving journey, do families have the money for a funeral if it is not prearranged? Is cremation a more financially feasible option? And, sometimes more to the point, is a funeral or memorial service worth the *bother*?

Here is my concern. If we view death as an inconvenience, a lamentable disruption in life, we often choose to move through the process as expeditiously as possible. In fact, the dying person may even be concerned that the funeral or memorial service will be a burden, a *bother*, for the surviving family members. You know, everyone is so busy these days! Just do something easy and get on with life. As if it were that easy.

The reality is this. The end-of-life ritual for a family or friend *is* a bother. And it should be! The surviving family and friends should *bother* to celebrate the life of the deceased. They should *bother* to confront the pain of loss. They should *bother* to recount the stories of a life lived. They should *bother* to give thanks for blessings shared. They should *bother* to support one another in their grief. They should *bother* to find meaning in the midst of despair. They should *bother* to find the courage to mourn and the hope to survive. Yes, ritual *is* worth the *bother*!

To Summarize...

- For many caregivers and care receivers, the terminating event of the caregiving journey is death. Hence, as with all other aspects of the journey, we need to proactively plan for that eventuality.

- We live in a death-averse society. Consequently, our fear of death often inhibits our ability to be present in the moment. We miss the opportunities and the possibilities afforded at the end of the road.

- Our attitudes about death and dying are informed and influenced by cultural, family, societal, and spiritual norms. Some influences serve to increase our death anxiety; others serve to mitigate our fear of death. We are wise to critically assess our attitudes about death and dying, modifying behaviors and attitudes that inhibit our ability to live fully.

- During times of significant loss such as death, we hunger for the familiar, for the known. We also long for a sense of community, continuity, and meaning. End-of-life rituals provide the needed and desired connections. Rituals evolve as society evolves, but the need for ritual is timeless. Always remember, rituals are worth the *bother*.

Chapter 22

A Caregiving Benediction

A benediction is a short invocation in which we ask for help, blessings, and guidance. Therefore, there is no better way to conclude our conversation about the journey of caregiving than with a benediction. We need all the help we can get as we care for each other! So, as the caregiving journey unfolds one step at a time, may we all be blessed in the following ways:

- May we have the courage to care for each other.

- May we feel companioned in the caregiving journey.

- May we have the wisdom to prepare to care.

- May we have sustaining faith to confront our fears.

- May we graciously offer *and* receive help.

- May we discover strength unimagined during times of loss.

- May we remain hopeful during the times of trial.

- May we recognize the sacred in the ordinary.

- May we engage the journey one step at a time.

- May we be grateful for the moment.

- May we humbly answer the call to care.

- May we listen well, love deeply, and live fully—all the way to the end of the road.

- May it be so.

Appendix A

Suggested Reading

Agronin, Marc E. 2011. *How We Age: A Doctor's Journey into the Heart of Growing Old.* Cambridge: Da Capo Press.

Ariès, Philippe. 1981. *The Hour of Our Death.* New York: Knopf.

Bonanno, George A. 2009. *The Other Side of Sadness: What the New Science of Bereavement Tells Us About Life After Loss.* New York: Basic Books.

Bridges, William. 2004. *Transitions: Making Sense of Life's Changes.* Cambridge: Da Capo Press.

Byock, Ira. 2004. *The Four Things That Matter Most: A Book About Living.* New York: Free Press.

De Hennezel, Marie. 1997. *Intimate Death: How the Dying Teach Us How to Live.* New York: A.A. Knopf.

De Hennezel, Marie. 2012. *The Art of Growing Old: Aging with Grace.* New York: Viking.

Doka, Kenneth J. 2009. *Counseling Individuals with Life-Threatening Illness.* New York: Springer Publishing Company.

Frankel, Richard, M., ed. 2003. *The Biopsychosocial Approach: Past, Present, Future.* New York: The University of Rochester Press.

Frankl, Viktor E. 1984. *Man's Search for Meaning: An Introduction to Logotherapy.* New York: Simon & Schuster.

Keller, W. Phillip. 1970. *A Shepherd Looks at Psalm 23.* Grand Rapids: Zondervan Publishing House.

Kübler-Ross, Elisabeth. 1969. *On Death and Dying.* New York: Macmillan.

Kushner, Harold S. 1981. *When Bad Things Happen to Good People.* New York: Avon Books.

Larson, Dale. 1993. *The Helper's Journey: Working with People Facing Grief, Loss, and Life-Threatening Illness*. Champaign: Research Press.

Lewis, C. S. 2001. *A Grief Observed*. San Francisco: HarperSanFrancisco.

McDaniel, Susan H., Jeri Hepworth, and William J. Doherty. 1992. *Medical Family Therapy*. New York: BasicBooks.

McGoldrick, Monica, Randy Gerson, and Sueli Petry. 2008. *Genograms: Assessment and Intervention*. New York: W.W. Norton & Company.

Meier, Diane E., Stephen L. Isaacs, and Robert G. Hughes. 2010. *Palliative Care: Transforming the Care of Serious Illness*. San Francisco: Jossey-Bass.

Papadatou, Danai. 2009. *In the Face of Death*. New York: Springer Publishing.

Pargament, Kenneth I. 1997. *The Psychology of Religion and Coping: Theory, Research, Practice*. New York: Guilford Press.

Quindlen, Anna. 2012. *Lots of Candles, Plenty of Cake*. New York: Random House.

Smith, Patricia. 2009. *To Weep for a Stranger: Compassion Fatigue in Caregiving*. Charleston: Createspace.

Sofka, Carla, Illene Noppe Cupit, and Kathleen Gilbert. 2012. *Dying, Death, and Grief in an Online Universe For Counselors and Educators*. New York: Springer Publishing.

Southwick, Steven M., and Dennis S. Charney. 2012. *Resilience: The Science of Mastering Life's Greatest Challenges*. New York: Cambridge University Press.

Spilka, Bernard, ed. 2003. *The Psychology of Religion*, 3rd ed. New York: Guilford Press.

Worden, James William. 2008. *Grief Counseling and Grief Therapy: A Handbook for the Mental Health Practitioner*. New York: Springer Publishing.

Yalom, Irvin D. 2008. *Staring at the Sun: Overcoming the Terror of Death*. San Francisco: Jossey-Bass.

Internet Resources

AARP (aarp.org)

AARP Caregiving Resource Center (aarp.org/home-family/caregiving)

Aging With Dignity (agingwithdignity.org)

Alzheimer's Association (alz.org)

American Pet Products Association (americanpetproducts.org)

American Psychological Association (apa.org)

California Healthcare Foundation (chcf.org)

Cardinal, LLC (cardinalife.com)

CaringBridge (caringbridge.org)

Center for Practical Bioethics (practicalbioethics.org)

Centers for Disease Control and Prevention (cdc.gov)

Coda Alliance (codaalliance.org)

Colorado State University (colostate.edu)

Family Caregiver Alliance (caregiver.org)

GenoPro (genopro.com)

Hospice Foundation of America (hospicefoundation.org)

Humane Society of the United States (humanesociety.org)

Lotsa Helping Hands (lotsahelpinghands.com)

MetLife Mature Market Institute (metlife.com/mmi)

National Hospice and Palliative Care Organization (nhpco.org)

National Institute on Aging (nia.nih.gov)

Social Security Administration (ssa.gov)

The Conversation Project (theconversationproject.org)

The Dougy Center (dougy.org)

US Census Bureau (census.gov)

CPSIA information can be obtained
at www.ICGtesting.com
Printed in the USA
FSHW021250311018
53450FS